Urodynamics, Neurourology and Pelvic Floor Dysfunctions

Series Editor

Marco Soligo
Obstetrics and Gynecology Department
Buzzi Hospital - University of Milan
Milan, Italy

The aim of the book series is to highlight new knowledge on physiopathology, diagnosis and treatment in the fields of pelvic floor dysfunctions, incontinence and neurourology for specialists (urologists, gynecologists, neurologists, pediatricians, physiatrists), nurses, physiotherapists and institutions such as universities and hospitals.

More information about this series at http://www.springer.com/series/13503

Gianfranco Lamberti • Donatella Giraudo
Stefania Musco

Editors

Suprapontine Lesions and Neurogenic Pelvic Dysfunctions

Assessment, Treatment and Rehabilitation

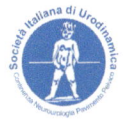

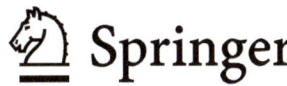

Editors
Gianfranco Lamberti
Neurorehabilitation Unit and Pelvic Floor
Dysfunction Rehabilitation Center
SS Trinità Hospital
Cuneo
Italy

Donatella Giraudo
Urology Department
San Raffaele Hospital
Milano
Italy

Stefania Musco
Department of Neurourology
Careggi University Hospital
Florence
Italy

ISSN 2510-4047   ISSN 2510-4055   (electronic)
Urodynamics, Neurourology and Pelvic Floor Dysfunctions
ISBN 978-3-030-29774-9   ISBN 978-3-030-29775-6   (eBook)
https://doi.org/10.1007/978-3-030-29775-6

This Springer imprint is published by the registered company Springer Nature Switzerland AG
The registered company address is: Gewerbestrasse 11, 6330 Cham, Switzerland

Foreword

Since 2015, Springer has published five volumes on functional pelvic floor hot topics under the auspices of the Italian Society of Urodynamics (SIUD). Our volumes always try to portray at best functional aspects in different clinical settings: oncology, male urology, genital prolapse, paediatrics, giving original and innovative perspectives in different backgrounds in an eclectic way.

The present volume fulfils our mission, looking at neurogenic pelvic floor dysfunctions from an original and, at the present time, still poorly investigated point of view: the suprapontine lesions. Since recent years, neurourologists have been focusing mainly on spinal cord lesions, developing high-level expertise in their understanding and management. More recently, also driven by the changing epidemiology of neurological disorders with an impact on pelvic floor functions, suprapontine lesions are increasingly becoming a matter of study. This book will offer an in-depth look on this topic from a multidisciplinary and multi-professional perspective, widening the scenario of potentially interested readers, spanning from neurourologists and clinicians devoted to urodynamics, to those operating in stroke units, including all the rehabilitation professional figures who will find an updated understanding of the set of problems many of their patients are involved with. The international faculty further guarantees an appealing experience with this book.

In the major interest of our patients, we do hope this volume will pique your interest.

Prof. Marco Soligo
Adjunct Professor in Urogynecology - University of Milan
President of the Italian Society of Urodynamics (SIUD)
Milan, Italy

Preface

If we wanted to choose an area of rehabilitation, the field in which we can find the most multicultural and interprofessional evolution, this could be indeed the rehabilitation of perineal and pelvic dysfunctions. Despite that, few are known about the role of pelvic rehabilitation in some specific neurological populations who potentially benefit on that. The purpose of this book is to provide a general introduction to the knowledge of pelvic disorders in people affected by suprapontine lesion. The book is addressed to professionals who are dealing with these types of illnesses for the first time as well as to those who are already experts and want to extend their knowledge and interests in this field.

The book takes its cue from the literature and gives more in-depth insights on the diagnosis and treatment of neurogenic urinary and bowel dysfunctions considering also the evolution of the functional imaging techniques in the last decades which has helped us to better understand the physiopathological differences and peculiarities of this subtype of neurological patients having suprapontine lesions and secondary pelvic dysfunctions. The interdisciplinary and multidisciplinary fields of actions involving doctors and health professionals (often with profoundly different backgrounds) are often still uncharted, but surely, it should tend towards an increasingly holistic view, in which overall components cannot be dissociable from the context. Furthermore, the relationships and networks between damage, brain function, bladder and intestinal behaviour are still poorly understood. Thus, the management of pelvic floor dysfunctions in such complex patients is a harder challenge to face compared to non-neurological or even in spinal cord-injured patients.

We hope that this book can open up ways of communication among different professionals by making this topic more accessible, often inexplicably confined (concerning the epidemiological impact and quality of life), to few specialized centres.

In order to make the material more friendly, we have tried to easily explain the various subtopics to be understandable even by professionals who are not specialists in neurourology. We hope we have succeeded in giving a reasonably exhaustive view of this area of its extensive and complex investigations and treatments, in such a way as to involve professionals of other specialties (e.g. rehabilitation, internal medicine, neurology) who often are involved in these pathologies.

After a general introduction on the neurophysiopathology of suprapontine lesions, the book is divided into chapters, each one concerning a specific subtopic including the diagnosis and treatment of the various pelvic dysfunctions among the different types of neurological suprapontine lesions. The influence of the clinical experience in the daily management of these problems is evident in the development and writing of the authors' contributions.

The main epidemiological aspects, always in relation to the patient with a suprapontine lesion, clinical evaluation of the perineum and the main reflexes, functional imaging of the central nervous system, urodynamic investigation and chronic pelvic pain are then taken into consideration. Particular attention has been paid to the rehabilitative aspects of bowel dysfunctions, often neglected in these neurological subpopulations compared to spinal cord injury patients. Again, also, two interesting but still poorly addressed arguments have been taken into account, namely, pelvic floor muscle training and sexual dysfunctions. The various chapters necessary for educational purposes are actually to be understood as inseparable moments of a unitary and continuous process.

The writing of this book would not have been possible without the tolerance and goodwill of many of our colleagues to whom we extend our gratitude. Finally, we are very grateful to our many patients who, despite the personal tragedy of brain damage, have made the development of our observations possible.

Milano, Italy   Donatella Giraudo
Florence, Italy   Stefania Musco
Piacenza, Italy   Gianfranco Lamberti

Contents

The Bladder, the Rectum and the Sphincters: Neural Pathways and Peripheral Control

1

Gianfranco Lamberti and Antonella Biroli

1.1 Introduction

Despite the fundamental contribution given by functional imaging in recent years, to date, the relationships between the different pathways in coordinating the alternation between the bladder-filling phase and the emptying phase have not yet been clarified nor, above all, which area should be considered as the "final decision maker" for activating micturition. The periaqueductal grey (PAG) and the pontine micturition centre (PMC) (Fig. 1.1), under physiological conditions with mutual influence, under the voluntary control of the prefrontal cortex (PFC) (Fig. 1.2), control the function. These three areas, in turn influenced by various afferents, coordinate the synchronisation between recruitment and inhibition of smooth and striated muscles [1–6] which regulate the behaviour of the bladder (the system's reservoir), the bladder neck and the urethra. The neural control is peripherally guaranteed by the parasympathetic sacral nerve (pelvic nerves), by the sympathetic thoracic lumbar nerve (hypogastric nerves) and by the sacral somatic nerve [pudendal nerve] [7, 8].

The importance of bladder control in controlling the homeostasis of the organism is guaranteed by the regular emptying of the bladder itself, which must be both safe and appropriate.

Processing the sensation of the bladder filling up is a cognitive element for maintaining equilibrium [9–11] which must determine finalised behaviours and consequent coherent motor activities [12].

The progression of the feeling of fullness begins with nerve signals whose frequency, intensity and unpleasantness increase proportionally to the bladder filling,

G. Lamberti (✉)
Neurorehabilitation Unit and Pelvic Floor Dysfunction Rehabilitation Center,
SS Trinità Hospital, Cuneo, Italy

A. Biroli
Neurological and Autonomic Dysfunction Rehabilitation Unit,
S.G. Bosco Hospital, Turin, Italy

© Springer Nature Switzerland AG 2020
G. Lamberti et al. (eds.), *Suprapontine Lesions and Neurogenic Pelvic Dysfunctions*, Urodynamics, Neurourology and Pelvic Floor Dysfunctions,
https://doi.org/10.1007/978-3-030-29775-6_1

1

Fig. 1.1 Cerebral and brainstem nuclei and pathways related to micturition and defecation. Abbreviations: *CC* Corpus callosum, *FNX* Fornix, *HY* Hypothalamus, *DLF* Fasciculus longitudinalis dorsalis, *PAG* Periaqueductal grey, *PBN* Parabrachial nucleus, *SOL* Nucleus solitarius. 1 = Pontine micturition centre (PMC). 2 = Kölliker-Fuse nucleus. 3 = Pontine continence centre (PCC)

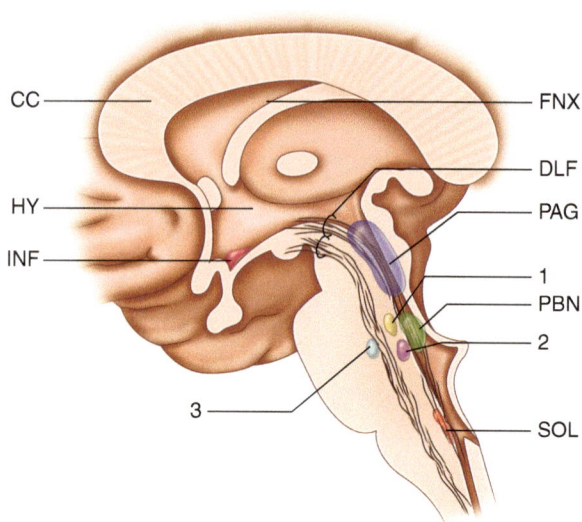

Fig. 1.2 Hippocampus, amygdala, subregions of prefrontal cortex and dorsal anterior cingulate cortex, cerebral areas associated with the control of the temporal and spatial appropriateness of social continence

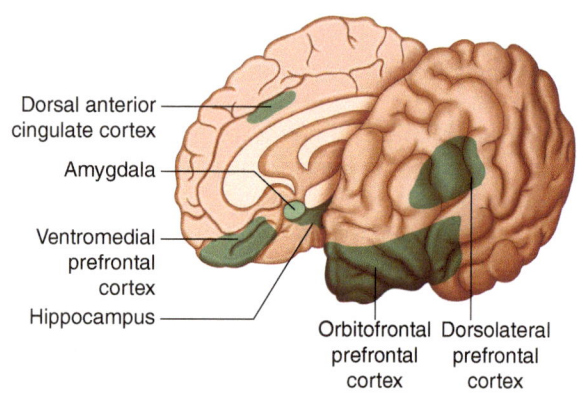

until the individual is obliged to urinate: the fullness cannot be maintained indefinitely and at some point the bladder must be emptied.

1.2   The Bladder Function

The filling and the emptying phase:

Urodynamic tests record the perception of the fullness level: the "first filling sensation" in healthy subjects (a sensation that is often not precisely perceptible, which often one does not pay attention to) occurs at about 40% of the total capacity of the detrusor; the International Continence Society (ICS) defines the "first desire to urinate as the sensation during a flow cystometry, which would lead the patient to urinate at the first opportune moment, although with the possibility of postponing further the emptying" [13] and usually refers to approximately 60% of the total

Fig. 1.3 Bladder filling, desire to void and behaviour

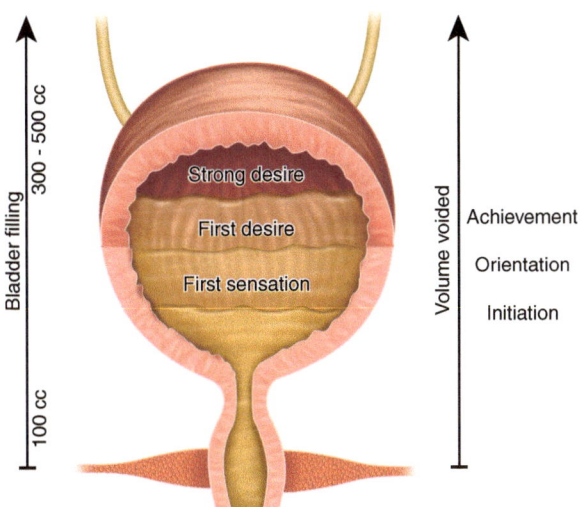

detrusor capacity. The "strong desire" to urinate is defined by ICS as "the persistent urge to urinate without the fear of the urine escaping" [13] (Fig. 1.3). These three conditions should be considered normal; the appearance of a "sudden and impelling desire to empty" (urgency) can instead be considered as a symptom of overactive bladder syndrome. People who report urinary urgency should, in any case, be considered in a non-physiological condition concerning the bladder function.

Under normal conditions, continence control allows the accumulation of urine, preventing emptying until the filling is complete.

The emptying phase only lasts for a short period of the complete behavioural cycle: considering how long the micturition can last and that it can be done six or seven times a day, the time dedicated to emptying does not exceed 1% of the total time [14].

Finally, the emptying occurs only if appropriate and the main criteria are social (adequate place and adequate time) and behavioural appropriateness (an adequate situation in order to avoid any embarrassment concerning the gesture) [15]. It is known that an attentional shift can influence the perception of the bladder-filling status, similarly to what occurs with the perception of pain, while a state of anxiety can increase the level of the desire to urinate, which only confirms how many psychological conditions may, in fact, alter the state of perception of the fullness of the bladder [14].

1.2.1   Spinal Cord Afferents

The afferent pathways reach the lower urinary tract through the pelvic, hypogastric nerves and the pudendal nerve stem [5, 14, 16, 17]: they are activated by the bladder distension and inhibit the detrusor parasympathetic system. Thanks to modern impregnation techniques it is possible to map first-level axons, coming from the peripheral areas, directed towards the lumbosacral posterior root ganglia (dorsal root ganglion, DRG) and to the terminations in the spinal cord, in order to then interpret their hypothetical role. The neurons from the detrusor wall project to the lumbar (T11–L2) and sacral (S2–S4) tracts and are responsible for controlling spinal reflex activity and for transmitting the perception of the need to urinate through the ascending pathways to the encephalic regions.

In men, it is possible to identify a dense nervous network ("sensory web") [4] widespread in the basal urothelial layer of the bladder [18–20] with some nerve endings projecting as far as the urothelium [21–23]; hence the medullary afferents are represented by two different types of fibres: myelinated fibres "A-δ" and small non-myelinated "C" fibres [24–28] (Fig. 1.4).

The lower threshold fibres ("A-δ") are myelinated (while non-myelinated fibres—"C" fibres—have higher thresholds) [4] and in most cases are sensitive to mechanical stimulation and respond to the bladder filling with a varying

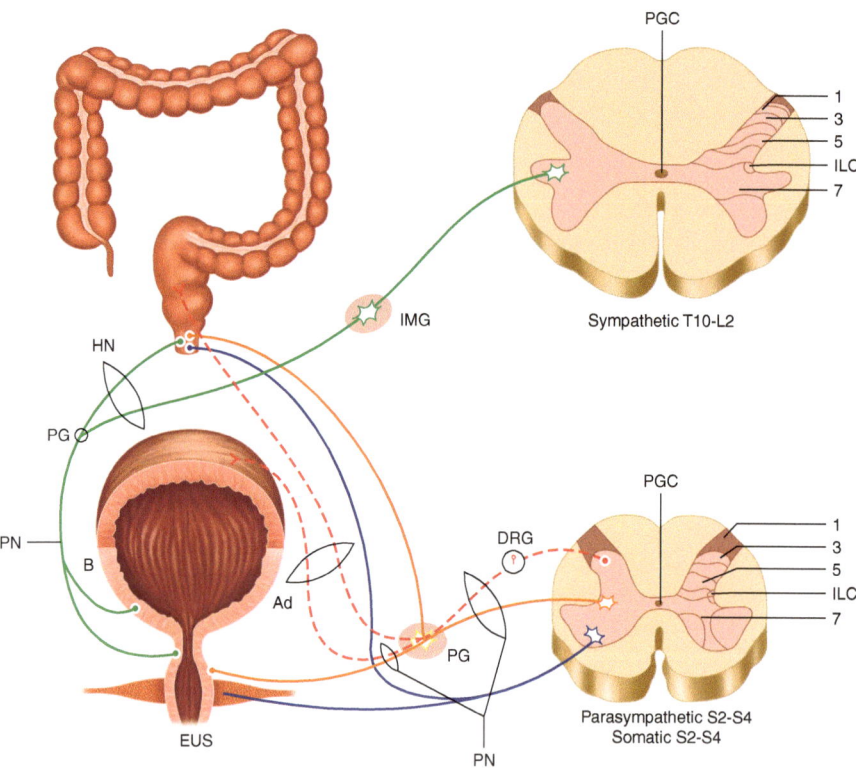

Fig. 1.4 Neural control of the lower urinary tract. Abbreviations: *PG* Pelvic ganglion, *IMG* Inferomesenteric ganglion, *HN* Hypogastric nerve, *PN* Pelvic nerve, *DRG* Dorsal root ganglion, *PGC* Posterior grey commissure, *ILC* Intermedio-lateral column: 1, 3, 5, 7 = Rexed laminae I, III, V, VII. Dotted line = Afferent pathways. Full line = Efferent pathways

volume sensitivity threshold, from normal filling to extreme distension. Both passive distension and active contraction activate fibres with larger diameters to convey information related to bladder filling in physiological conditions [16]. The fibres with smaller diameters can normally be called "silent", since they do not operate with bladder distension alone, except with large volumes; also found in the intestine, they are instead able to convey information from intra-luminal stimuli of a chemoceptive nature such as saline hypertonicity or that of a thermal nature [29, 30] sensitising themselves in pathological conditions (neuropathic or inflammatory ones) and determining the sensation of urgency or visceral pain.

In addition to the intrinsic characteristics of the detrusor smooth muscle, the fill-ing phase is made possible by the inhibition of the parasympathetic efferent path-ways [3] and by the sympathetic system with the activation of the sphincter function [31, 32]. Bladder adaptation allows an intra-bladder pressure with low values with a volume below the threshold of the desire to urinate.

The afferent bladder fibres project to the posterior horn of the sacral cord [33–37]. These neurons possess two interesting characteristics: they project directly to the PAG and the Rexed laminae V, VII and X [38, 39], regions containing parasympa-thetic interneurons and parasympathetic dendrites [38, 39].

This "direct" connection with the PAG [35, 40] (and not with the PMC) is typical of human, cat and dog and would allow control of the bladder filling without its perception (the latter guaranteed by the thalamus). Only reaching a certain filling level would determine the passage of information between the PAG and the PMC (and therefore its awareness) and the potential choice of voiding [37].

The intraspinal neurons identified as involved in spinal segmental reflexes [41–47] with excitatory and inhibitory synaptic connections [48–51] are located in the Rexed laminae I, V and VII and the posterior grey commissure [52–58] (Fig. 1.4).

The afferent pathways of the pelvic area originating from the urethra, the ure-thral sphincter and the neuromuscular pelvic spindles present an essentially over-lapping pattern of endings [59] and this arrangement presumably coordinates the pelvic floor muscles (PFM) and the sphincteric function during micturition and defecation [60].

The overlap between the dendritic afferents from the detrusor and the urethra on the posterior horns and on the posterior grey commissure indicates that these regions are the most important routes for receiving information from the peripheral area: these are probably essential sites for the visceral-somatic integration which may represent a fundamental element in coordinating the detrusor function and the sphincter activity, which in fact have a similar dendritic pattern [33]. In summary, during the entire filling phase, the sensation of the detrusor being full is conveyed, thanks to first-order neurons, by the pelvic and hypogastric nerves [5, 16] while the hypogastric nerves and the pudendal nerve convey the sensory information from the neck of the bladder and the urethra [4].

Some spinal interneurons connect with the bladder afferents [52, 54, 55], trans-mitting signals through the ascending sensory pathway and reaching, after a partial decussation [35], mainly the gracile nucleus (which conveys the nociceptive sensitivity to the thalamus and the cortex), the PMC and the PAG [10], that is in turn connected with numerous other brain areas [61–63] through third-order neurons [63, 64]. There is a second ascending pathway to the gracile nucleus from the pelvic organs and subsequently to the thalamus for transmitting nociceptive impulses [65].

1.2.2   Spinal Cord Efferents

The sympathetic preganglionic system is located medially and laterally in the lumbar spinal cord segments, the external urethral sphincter motor neurons in Onuf's nucleus and the parasympathetic preganglionic neurons in the sacral cord segments.

The preganglionic cholinergic efferent neurons reach the pelvic plexus ganglia and the detrusor wall. The axons originate from the sacral parasympathetic nucleus from S2 to S4, and have synaptic connections with the pelvic ganglia as well as with the small ganglia on the detrusor wall which release acetylcholine. Nicotinic receptors mediate postsynaptic activation: postganglionic axons run for a short distance in the pelvic nerves and have terminations in the detrusor wall where they release acetylcholine which induces the contraction of the smooth muscle fibres. Muscarinic receptors mediate this postganglionic stimulation; there are two subtypes of muscarinic receptors, M2 and M3, in the detrusor: although M2 receptors are more numerous, subtype M3 is specific for the contractions of the detrusor [66, 67].

During the filling phase, the whole set of active afferents and efferents, under physiological conditions, allows continence to be maintained, thanks to the presence of urethral reflexes known as a whole as "guarding reflex" [4, 10, 14, 68–70]. In the pelvic-hypogastric component of the "guarding reflex", the parasympathetic innervation of the detrusor is inhibited while at the same time the smooth (internal urethral sphincter, through the hypogastric nerve) and striated components (external urethral sphincter, through the pudendal nerve) are active. The pelvic-pudendal component of the reflex, similarly active, under normal conditions, in the occasion of increases in intra-abdominal pressure (cough, laughter and physical activity), through the action of glutamatergic pathways and N-methyl-D-aspartate receptors (NMDA) with the release of acetylcholine, is responsible for the anticipatory contraction of the external urethral sphincter.

Unlike what occurs in animals, where the sympathetic lumbar nerve contributes mainly to inhibiting the detrusor's smooth muscle and to contracting the bladder neck [71, 72], in man there could be a control exercised specifically during the filling phase by the activation of the dorsal portion of the anterior cingulate cortex (dACC) (Fig. 1.2) and of the surrounding sensory-motor areas, together with the action of the supplementary motor area, which is active when PFM and urethral striated sphincter contract [73–77].

Similar control is exercised from an area at the dorsal-lateral pontine tegmentum, known as "pontine continence centre" (PCC) (Fig. 1.1), which facilitates the reflex activity of the sphincters [7, 10, 64, 78–88]. This area would receive signals directly from Onuf's nucleus and its stimulation, activated via the spinal reflex pathway by sub-threshold afferent impulses coming from the bladder, would contribute to activating the "guarding reflex" [33].

The contraction of the PFM simultaneously with a strong desire to urinate activates the PCC, particularly just before beginning the micturition, and its electrical stimulation activates the motor neurons of the external urethral sphincter (EUS) and induces its contraction [2, 78, 89].

The contraction of the EUS activates afferent fibres of the pudendal nerve which suppress the reflex activity of the bladder [90] by inhibiting the parasympathetic preganglionic neurons and the interneurons which belong to the micturition reflex pathway [91, 92], promoting urinary continence [78, 93].

Reaching a certain critical level of distension of the detrusor wall provoked by the mechanoreceptors [42, 84, 92] causes the "switch" from the "off" phase of filling to the "on" phase of emptying. This process involves a circuit which conveys the bladder afferents to the midbrain and the pons and is regulated by the spinal-medulla oblongata emptying reflex [69].

In reality, emptying the bladder, under physiological conditions, involves the supraspinal centres and pathways [94, 95]: in fact, the presence of an exclusively "reflex" circuit would cause an "involuntary" emptying, with consequent urinary incontinence, once it reaches a specific filling volume. This is what happens in the child; in the adult, under physiological conditions, however, the reflex is strictly controlled by the pons and by the brain, and the decision to urinate, fundamentally crucial in human behaviour, is usually taken only at the appropriate time and place. It is, therefore, the result of a combination of different physiological, emotional and behavioural factors.

1.2.3   The Periaqueductal Grey and the Pontine Micturition Centre

Several functional brain imaging studies have shown how the PAG is activated during the filling phase [61, 63, 64, 96–98] and can, therefore, be considered to all effects the integrating centre between different afferent and efferent circuits of the bladder [99, 100], as it is able to excite or inhibit the bladder activity [101–105], since the GABA is the mediator involved in these inhibitory mechanisms [106].

There is now a broad consensus on the role of the PAG as the structure which integrates somatic and autonomic sensory afferents with emotional components in order to coordinate the reaction to stress, reproductive behaviour [107], aggression, sense of defence, response to visceral pain [108, 109] and maternal behaviour [110], and this has determined its definition as part of the "emotional motor system" [111].

The afferents from the pelvic organs reach the mesencephalic PAG through the connections with the pontine centres [112]: reflexively [demonstrated by electrical stimulation] [113] the PAG determines the emptying of the bladder, but under normal physiological conditions its activity is conditioned by the information that allows the person to judge whether the micturition is appropriate based on place and time.

Similar control is also likely for defecation and sexual activity [114].

In the animal it was possible to record single neuronal units of PAG, which show different activation patterns: "tonic" and "phasic" filling neurons, which are, respectively, partially or entirely inhibited during detrusor contractions, and "tonic" and "phasic" neurons which are active exclusively during the detrusor emptying phase [115].

Neurons also appear to be distributed, according to their activity, in different areas of the PAG, for that matter connected by interneurons [113].

In addition to the circuits which interface the PAG and the PMC and the spinal pathways coordinating the detrusor contraction with the relaxation of the sphincter during the emptying one, another significant element is represented by the fact that the bladder afferents end in the central portion of the PAG, while the PMC efferents originate from more lateral portions of the PAG itself: these connections modulate the "switch" between the emptying and the filling phases to trigger the emptying or to maintain continence [116].

The numerous connections of the PAG with the superior areas are the neuronal substrate for the control of the temporal and spatial appropriateness of social continence from the brain (dorsal anterior cingulate cortex, insula, amygdala and ventromedial prefrontal cortex) [117] (Fig. 1.2).

The PAG, in turn, projects caudally to the PMC (also known as Barrington's nucleus) (Fig. 1.1) allowing information about the level of fullness of the bladder and processes the superior influences responsible for the voiding reflex.

The PMC is located in the pontine tegmentum near the locus coeruleus (LC) [4, 37]; the importance of this area located in the pons concerning bladder control was first demonstrated in the cat [1] and subsequently also confirmed in other species [118, 119], and finally functional imaging studies have confirmed the activation of the dorsal pontine regions in humans at the beginning of voluntary micturition [120–122].

The PMC projects to the parasympathetic bladder motor neurons of the sacral cord (Onuf's nucleus): the mutual coordination between sphincter and detrusor is determined by the fact that the PMC activates not only the glutamatergic fibres facilitating the parasympathetic sacral preganglionic nucleus [123] but also the GABAergic and glycinergic inhibitory interneurons which reduce the activity of Onuf's nucleus with the consequent inhibition of the urethral sphincter when the detrusor contracts. There is also evidence of projections from the PMC to the locus coeruleus (LC) [124–126]; as the main noradrenergic centre of the brain, the LC sends collateral projections to the entire CNS, including the cerebral cortex [127], modulating neuronal activity [128] and displacement of the focus of attention due to new stimuli in respect of the ongoing activities: in this case an increase in attention to visceral stimulation is determined, which "would prepare" the organism for an adequate emptying.

1.2.4   The Cortical Control

The prefrontal cortex is responsible for the programming of the appropriate micturition behaviour, the expression of the personality of the person and his/her proper social behaviour.

In modulating these activities, the midbrain parabrachial nucleus [129] (Fig. 1.1), the ventromedial cord area [130], the midbrain [116] and the pontine tegmentum [131] would also intervene, by all providing, with different degrees and ways, some setting level for a correct "switch" to the emptying phase. The midbrain parabrachial nucleus would also be responsible for processing abnormal stimuli in case of hyperactivity of the detrusor.

The insula, considered the seat of the interoception, i.e. the place where the physiological sensations of the entire organism, including visceral sensitivity, are processed, also contributes to modulating the responses; in this case the afferents are conveyed through small-diameter fibres in the spinal cord through the Rexed lamina I, exactly as occurs for the bladder afferents (Fig. 1.4). The Rexed lamina I neurons project to the thalamus and the lobe of the insula; processing visceral afferents is therefore closely associated with and conditioned by affective and motivational aspects.

The cerebellum [132, 133] and the hypothalamus are also involved in subcortical modulation patterns. The caudal hypothalamus is activated in relation to the filling-emptying phases of the bladder [134, 135]; in the animal, the stimulation of its anterior portion results in the assumption of the typical posture for micturition or defecation [136]. Together with the PAG, the hypothalamus can activate the PMC, thus eliciting the voiding reflex [97, 98].

The cortex of the anterior cingulate gyrus (Brodmann area 32), an area associated with the motivational component of the gesture, that can be considered to all effects the "limbic" motor cortex, participates in the bladder control. The basal ganglia control micturition in a mainly inhibitory role [137] by physiologically activating the globus pallidus during the bladder filling [96]. Dopamine controls the urinary reflex (with an inhibitory action through D1 receptors and a facilitating one through D2 receptors) and by GABA (by inhibitory action) [138]. Dopamine released by the substantia nigra and by the striatum nucleus activates the D1-GABAergic dopamine direct pathway which inhibits the globus pallidus and the substantia nigra reticulata and also inhibits the urinary reflex through the collateral GABAergic pathways to the PAG [139].

Co-activation of the insular lobe and the cortex of the anterior cingulate gyrus during the filling phase is frequently detectable in functional imaging studies [140] and often occurs during activation of the attentional state by the sympathetic system. Activation of the right PMC, insular lobe and dorsal portion of the anterior cingulate gyrus have been correlated in healthy subjects to the degree of bladder filling and to the desire to urinate normally.

The limbic system as a whole has close connections with the prefrontal cortex, suggesting that emotional behaviour and cognitive processes are closely linked [141].

PET studies demonstrate the deactivation of the medial prefrontal cortex, which coincides with the bladder-filling phase, while it is activated during the emptying one. The presence of a "normal" filling sensation, therefore, would ensure continence, also when not reaching the level of a conscious stimulus.

When the decision to empty the bladder is made, the prefrontal cortex, the insular lobe, the hypothalamus, the PAG and the PMC are activated: the activation of the PMC is the final efferent brain effect, and in a healthy subject it determines the transmission of the information to void the bladder to the spinal cord sacral segments.

1.3   The Bowel Function

Faecal continence and defecation are intimately connected and dependent on neurological control.

It is commonly accepted that the "normal" frequency of intestinal emptying varies between a minimum of three bowel movements a week and a maximum of three times a day [142]. The number of defecations is affected by several factors: psychological (anxiety) [143–145], organic [pain when defecating] [146], habit or need to postpone the evacuation, posture taken while defecating, colic transit speed and stool volume. The food intake increases peristalsis in the transverse and descending colon, and this occurs with a double-temporal peak, the first at 10–50 min from the food intake and the second at 70–90 min.

The "motor" activity of the colon is increased upon awakening [147] and after meals [148, 149].

The study of transit times has shown a duration of the passage in the colon of about 72 h on average, and the progression occurs thanks to the low-amplitude contractions (low-amplitude propagated contractions: LAPC) which occur 50–100 times a day, and to the high-amplitude ones (HAPC, high-amplitude propagated contractions) which occur 5–6 times a day in the adult [149, 150].

The arrival of the material (solid, liquid, gaseous) in the rectum activates through the pressure receptors present in PFM the recto-anal inhibitory reflex (RAIR) and the sampling of material in the anal canal.

In the case of complete control of the continence mechanisms, which, once reached, effectively allows to counter the need induced by the arrival of faecal material in the rectum, and in case of an inconvenient place or time for defecating or in case of the desire to postpone the act, PFM contraction allows postponing defecation [151].

At the moment when the decision to defecate is taken, with a correct diaphragmatic expiratory thrust, the anorectal angle becomes horizontal and the faecal material is expelled [152]. The normal condition is restored with the closing reflex [153].

The gastrointestinal functions are controlled by a neuronal network composed of about 500,000 neurons, distributed in the myenteric plexus and the submucosal plexus [154], which together constitute the enteric nervous system (ENS). The ENS includes different types of functionally distinct enteric neurons [primary intrinsic afferents, afferent and efferent interneurons, excitatory and inhibitory motor neurons], all synaptically bound together in neural circuits that regulate all reflexes occurring in the digestive tract, including those which regulate peristalsis [155].

This highly integrated neural system, located with the two myenteric and submucosal plexus systems in the intestinal tract wall and extended along its entire length, is considered the "brain in the gut", i.e. a nervous system able to control the various functions even when isolated anatomically from the CNS and from the peripheral nervous system (PNS).

The network that regulates the filling phase and the emptying phase of the distal colon depends primarily on this, through the proximodistal [but also distoproximal] propulsion [156] of the colic content and the defecation, thanks to the relaxation of the anal sphincter system [157].

This neural circuit belongs only and exclusively to the enteric tract, while the spinal and supraspinal control systems substantially overlap with those of the bladder system.

Obviously, in addition to ENS, which should be considered to all intents as the intrinsic innervation of the gastrointestinal tract, the sympathetic, parasympathetic and somatic systems regulate the gastrointestinal functions.

The sensory afferents, which activate the inhibition or recruitment of the smooth or striated muscle of the anal sphincter complex, come mainly from the rectum that has to guarantee a continuous compliance "reservoir" function and from the "sampling" area of the anorectal junction, tasked with the recognition of the faecal material.

The afferents to the sacral metamers are conveyed by sympathetic and parasympathetic nerves (splanchnic nerves, pelvic nerves and vagus nerve) and by somatic nerves (pudendal nerve) and reach the posterior horns located in the Rexed lamina I [158] (Fig. 1.4). The convergence of visceral somatic afferents allows explaining the phenomenon of "referred pain" (pain caused by a viscera section and perceived in a body area with sensory afferents which reach the same cord levels of the bowels) and of "cross sensitisation" between the different pelvic organs [159].

Anal sensitivity is conveyed by the lower rectal branch of the pudendal nerve. The cranial anal canal is rich in nerve endings (corpuscles of Krause for cold, of Golgi-Mazzoni for pressure, of Meissner for tactile sensitivity) [160, 161] while special afferents would transmit the temperature of the rectum.

The somatic spinal pathways (spinothalamic tract) reach the gracile nucleus and transmit information concerning the tactile sensitivity of the perineal area.

The processing of information following the distension of the rectal wall on arrival of the faecal bolus and the resulting stretch is allowed by the non-myelinated "C" fibres present in the rectal wall [162], and the specialised components for sensory-mechanical transduction (sensitive to the distension and contraction of the surrounding musculature) are in the myenteric ganglia of the rectum. There are various populations of afferent fibres which allow modulating the information about the distension of the walls: some transmit physiological information which enables the propulsion of the bolus, others are activated only above a certain threshold and contribute to inducing the nociceptive stimulus, and some others (usually "silent") are triggered exclusively during inflammatory phenomena [159].

Myelinated "Aδ" fibres provide the evocation and control of RAIR and the recto-anal excitatory reflex (RAER) in the mucosa [163].

The peripheral sympathetic afferents too are conveyed towards the Rexed lamina I, from which they project mainly non-myelinated "C" fibres towards the sympathetic thoracolumbar system and from here, through the ascending pathways, towards the centres of the brainstem (PMC, PAG and midbrain parabrachial nucleus); they subsequently reach different areas of signal processing of the autonomous nervous system (ANS), such as the solitary tract nucleus (STN), the hypothalamus and the amygdala [164–166].

The PAG and the STN moreover receive parasympathetic afferents which are also conveyed to the hypothalamus and amygdala [167], ensuring an optimal integration between the two systems. Coordination between activities of the proximal and the distal gastrointestinal tracts, together with the one between the sigmoid-rectal tract and the bladder, is guaranteed by the PMC, thanks to its relations with the sacral parasympathetic system and the motor nucleus of the vagus nerve [128, 168]. Its projections to the locus coeruleus activate neuronal circuits which govern attention and shifting of the attentional focus towards new stimuli in respect of activities already in progress [128]: in this case, as occurs with micturition, the perception of rectal filling leads to an increase in attention towards the visceral stimulus, which therefore "would prepare" the organism for an adequate rectal emptying [169].

Gastrointestinal motility and gastric secretion can be modulated by the Kölliker-Fuse (Fig. 1.1) nucleus or pneumotaxic centre and by the paraventricular nucleus (PVN) through either the cerebellum vestibular or the cerebellum hypothalamic pathways [170]. These connections would also explain the activation of the alert status together with the increase of colic transit which occurs in response to stress [171]: in this case the production of oxytocin and vasopressin (which are released by the posterior pituitary) and of the corticotropin-releasing hormone (corticotropin-releasing factor—CRF) by PVN, which also projects to the LC, increases.

The PMC too is involved in colonic function [172], guaranteeing its activity together with that of the vesicoureteral apparatus, and also ensuring, through the nucleus of the vagus nerve, the synergic activity of proximal and distal intestinal segments. Analogously as happens for the bladder the distension of the colon can activate the PMC, with a consequent increase in the colon's motility.

In addition to visceral afferents of lumbosacral origin, various encephalic, mesencephalic and brainstem projections reach the PMC, thus confirming the neuroanatomical integration between the colic function and different emotional and behavioural components.

Some pathways ascending from the Rexed lamina I directly reach the medial thalamus and from here the dACC, an area associated with the emotional aspects of pain perception; moreover, the facilitating and inhibitory pathways reach the Rexed lamina I neurons directly from the brainstem and from the LC, thus guaranteeing an even more complex level of processing the visceral afferents.

Vagal, cholinergic preganglionic fibres originate in the brainstem (the dorsal motor nucleus of the vagus nerve) [162, 173] and control the neurons of the myenteric plexus [174].

Preganglionic neurons controlling the parasympathetic innervation of the distal colon are in the lumbosacral cord (S1–S4 levels in the intermedio-lateral column) (Fig. 1.4): they are smaller than the preganglionic neurons which innervate the bladder [16], from which they are separated, and reach the colon with two pathways, directly innervating the postganglionic neurons of the myenteric plexus or innervating the postganglionic neurons in the hypogastric plexus ganglia [175] which in turn reach the colon through the rectal nerves: this would ensure a double-parasympathetic control of the colon, given that enteric neurons are present both in the spinal cord and in the pelvic ganglia. Parasympathetic innervation is fundamentally crucial for colon motility, in particular during defecation: any damage leads to constipation.

Sympathetic preganglionic neurons which innervate the gastrointestinal tract originate from the thoracic and lumbar spinal cord. In particular, the innervation of the colon is predominantly ensured by the L2–L5 levels which have an inhibitory action of the intestinal mobility, mediated by the myenteric plexus, and an excitatory one of the sphincter activity [176]. Preganglionic neurons are cholinergic and activate postganglionic neurons within the superior and the lower mesenteric ganglion; sympathetic and parasympathetic postganglionic neurons are both present in the pelvic ganglia: the crosstalk between the two systems guarantees the perfect neuronal integration of the system [177, 178].

The sacral plexus innervates the distal colon and the rectum with a network globally in common with the lower urinary tract [71, 179], which is similar to that guaranteed by the vagus nerve on the proximal tract; a substantial difference to bear in mind is the presence of fibres that carry the nociceptive message in the pelvic afferents (and not in the vagal ones).

The primary motor cortex is connected to the sacral motor nucleus of the pelvic floor muscles (Onuf's nucleus, the site of voluntary recruitment control): here, separated areas control urethral sphincter and external anal sphincter function.

Finally, defecation is the consequence of a reflex activated by the distension of the rectum. Emptying, in a substantially similar manner to what occurs for the bladder, in the adult is controlled by the spinal and supra-spinal centres.

References

1. Barrington F. The effect of lesions of the hind- and mid-brain on micturition in the cat. Q J Exp Physiol. 1925;15:81–102.
2. Kuru M. Nervous control of micturition. Physiol Rev. 1965;45:425–94.
3. de Groat WC, Booth AM, Yoshimura N. Neurophysiology of micturition and its modification in animal models of human disease. In: Maggi CA, editor. The autonomic nervous system. London: Harwood Academic Publishers; 1993. p. 227–89.
4. Fowler CJ, Griffiths D, de Groat WC. The neural control of micturition. Nat Rev Neurosci. 2008;9:453–66.

 5. Birder L, Blok B, Burnstock G, et al. Committee 3: Neural Control. In: Abrams P, Cardozo L, Wagg A, Wein A, editors. Incontinence. 6th International Consultation on Incontinence, Tokyo 2016. Paris: ICUD-ICS; 2017.
 6. Fry CH, Kanai AJ, Roosen A, et al. Cell biology. In: Abrams P, Cardozo L, Khoury S, Wein A, editors. Incontinence, vol. 4. Paris, France: Health Publications, Ltd; 2009. p. 113–66.
 7. de Groat WC, Wickens C. Organization of the neural switching circuitry underlying reflex micturition. Acta Physiol (Oxf). 2013;207(1):66–84.
 8. Arya NG, Weissbart SJ. Central control of micturition in women: brain-bladder pathways in continence and urgency urinary incontinence. Clin Anat. 2017;30(3):373–84.
 9. Critchley HD, Mathias CJ, Josephs O, et al. Human cingulate cortex and autonomic control: converging neuroimaging and clinical evidence. Brain. 2003;126:2139–52.
10. Mayer EA, Naliboff BD, Craig AD. Neuroimaging of the brain-gut axis: from basic understanding to treatment of functional GI disorders. Gastroenterology. 2006;131: 1925–42.
11. Lane RD, Wager TD. The new field of brain-body medicine: what have we learned and where are we headed? NeuroImage. 2009;47:1135–40.
12. Fowler CJ, Griffiths DJ. A decade of functional brain imaging applied to bladder control. Neurourol Urodyn. 2010;29:49–55.
13. Haylen BT, de Ridder D, Freeman RM, et al. An International Urogynecological Association (IUGA)/International Continence Society (ICS) joint report on the terminology for female pelvic floor dysfunction. Int Urogynecol J. 2010;21:5–26.
14. Fowler CJ. Integrated control of lower urinary tract—clinical perspective. Br J Pharmacol. 2006;147(Suppl 2):S14–24.
15. Griffiths D. Neural control of micturition in humans: a working model. Nat Rev Urol. 2015;12(12):695–705.
16. Janig W, Morrison JF. Functional properties of spinal visceral afferents supplying abdominal and pelvic organs, with special emphasis on visceral nociception. Prog Brain Res. 1986;67:87–114.
17. de Groat WC, Yoshimura N. Afferent nerve regulation of bladder function in health and disease. Handb Exp Pharmacol. 2009;194:91–138.
18. Gosling JA, Dixon JS. Sensory nerves in the mammalian urinary tract. An evaluation using light and electron microscopy. J Anat. 1974;117:133–44.
19. Gabella G. The structural relations between nerve fibres and muscle cells in the urinary bladder of the rat. J Neurocytol. 1995;24:159–71.
20. Gabella G, Davis C. Distribution of afferent axons in the bladders of rats. J Neurocytol. 1998;27:141–55.
21. Birder LA. Vanilloid receptor expression suggests a sensory role for urinary bladder epithelial cells. Proc Natl Acad Sci U S A. 2001;98:13396–401.
22. Birder L. Role of the urothelium in bladder function. Scand J Urol Nephrol Suppl. 2004;215:48–53.
23. Wiseman OJ. The ultrastructure of bladder lamina propria nerves in healthy subjects and patients with detrusor hyperreflexia. J Urol. 2002;168:2040–5.
24. Sengupta JN, Gebhart GF. Mechanosensitive properties of pelvic nerve afferent fibers innervating the urinary bladder of the rat. J Neurophysiol. 1994;72:2420–30.
25. Shea VK, Cai R, Crepps B, et al. Sensory fibers of the pelvic nerve innervating the Rat's urinary bladder. J Neurophysiol. 2000;84:1924–33.
26. Kanai A, Wyndaele JJ, Andersson KE, et al. Researching bladder afferents-determining the effects of beta(3)-adrenergic receptor agonists and botulinum toxin type-A. Neurourol Urodyn. 2011;30:684–91.
27. Habler HJ, Janig W, Koltzenburg M. Receptive properties of myelinated primary afferents innervating the inflamed urinary bladder of the cat. J Neurophysiol. 1993;69:395–405.
28. Gillespie JI, van Koeveringe GA, de Wachter SG, de Vente J. On the origins of the sensory output from the bladder: the concept of afferent noise. BJU Int. 2009;103:1324–33.

29. Habler HJ, Janig W, Koltzenburg M. Activation of unmyelinated afferent fibres by mechanical stimuli and inflammation of the urinary bladder in the cat. J Physiol. 1990;425:545–62.
30. Fall M, Lindström S, Mazieres L. A bladder-to-bladder cooling reflex in the cat. J Physiol. 1990;427:281–300.
31. de Groat WC, Lalley PM. Reflex firing in the lumbar sympathetic outflow to activation of vesical afferent fibres. J Physiol. 1972;226:289–309.
32. de Groat WC, Theobald RJ. Reflex activation of sympathetic pathways to vesical smooth muscle and parasympathetic ganglia by electrical stimulation of vesical afferents. J Physiol. 1976;259:223–37.
33. Thor KB, de Groat WC. Neural control of the female urethral and anal rhabdosphincters and pelvic floor muscles. Am J Physiol Regul Integr Comp Physiol. 2010;299:R416–38.
34. Holstege G. Micturition and the soul. J Comp Neurol. 2005;493:15–20.
35. Klop EM, Mouton LJ, Kuipers R, et al. Neurons in the lateral sacral cord of the cat project to periaqueductal grey, but not to thalamus. Eur J Neurosci. 2005;21:2159–66.
36. Beckel JM, Holstege G. Neurophysiology of the lower urinary tract. Handb Exp Pharmacol. 2011;8:149–69.
37. Holstege G. The emotional motor system and micturition control. Neurourol Urodyn. 2010;29:42–8.
38. Morgan C, Nadelhaft I, de Groat WC. The distribution of visceral primary afferents from the pelvic nerve to Lissauer's tract and the spinal gray matter and its relationship to the sacral parasympathetic nucleus. J Comp Neurol. 1981;201:415–40.
39. Steers WD, Ciambotti J, Etzel B, et al. Alterations in afferent pathways from the urinary bladder of the rat in response to partial urethral obstruction. J Comp Neurol. 1991;310:401–10.
40. Van der Horst V, Mouton L, Blok B, et al. Somatotopical organization of input from the lumbosacral cord to the periaqueductal gray in the cat; possible implications for aggressive and defensive behavior, micturition, and lordosis. J Comp Neurol. 1996;376:361–85.
41. Blok B, Holstege G. The pontine micturition center in rat receives direct lumbosacral input. An ultrastructural study. Neurosci Lett. 2000;282:29–32.
42. de Groat WC, Araki I, Vizzard MA, et al. Developmental and injury induced plasticity in the micturition reflex pathway. Behav Brain Res. 1998;92:127–40.
43. McMahon SB, Morrison JF. Spinal neurones with long projections activated from the abdominal viscera of the cat. J Physiol. 1982;322:1–20.
44. Ding YQ, Zheng HX, Gong LW, et al. Direct projections from the lumbosacral spinal cord to Barrington's nucleus in the rat: a special reference to micturition reflex. J Comp Neurol. 1997;389:149–60.
45. Holstege G, Mouton LJ. Central nervous system control of micturition. Int Rev Neurobiol. 2003;56:123–45.
46. Birder LA, Roppolo JR, Erickson VL, et al. Increased c-fos expression in spinal lumbosacral projection neurons and preganglionic neurons after irritation of the lower urinary tract in the rat. Brain Res. 1999;834:55–65.
47. Thor KB, Morgan C, Nadelhaft I, et al. Organization of afferent and efferent pathways in the pudendal nerve of the female cat. J Comp Neurol. 1989;288:263–79.
48. Araki I, de Groat WC. Unitary excitatory synaptic currents in preganglionic neurons mediated by two distinct groups of interneurons in neonatal rat sacral parasympathetic nucleus. J Neurophysiol. 1996;76:215–26.
49. Araki I, de Groat WC. Developmental synaptic depression underlying reorganization of visceral reflex pathways in the spinal cord. J Neurosci. 1997;17:8402–7.
50. Miura A, Kawatani M, de Groat WC. Excitatory synaptic currents in lumbosacral parasympathetic preganglionic neurons evoked by stimulation of the dorsal commissure. J Neurophysiol. 2003;89:382–9.
51. Morgan CW, de Groat WC, Felkins LA, et al. Intracellular injection of neurobiotin or horseradish peroxidase reveals separate types of preganglionic neurons in the sacral parasympathetic nucleus of the cat. J Comp Neurol. 1993;331:161–82.

52. Nadelhaft I, Vera PL, Card JP, et al. Central nervous system neurons labelled following the injection of pseudorabies virus into the rat urinary bladder. Neurosci Lett. 1992;143:271–4.

53. Nadelhaft I, Vera PL. Central nervous system neurons infected by pseudorabies virus injected into the rat urinary bladder following unilateral transection of the pelvic nerve. J Comp Neurol. 1995;359:443–56.

54. Nadelhaft I, Vera PL. Neurons in the rat brain and spinal cord labeled after pseudorabies virus injected into the external urethral sphincter. J Comp Neurol. 1996;375:502–17.

55. Nadelhaft I, Vera PL. Separate urinary bladder and external urethral sphincter neurons in the central nervous system of the rat: simultaneous labeling with two immunohistochemically distinguishable pseudorabies viruses. Brain Res. 2001;903:33–44.

56. Vizzard MA, Erickson VL, Card JP, et al. Transneuronal labeling of neurons in the adult rat brainstem and spinal cord after injection of pseudorabies virus into the urethra. J Comp Neurol. 1995;355:629–40.

57. Sugaya K, Roppolo JR, Yoshimura N, et al. The central neural pathways involved in micturition in the neonatal rat as revealed by the injection of pseudorabies virus into the urinary bladder. Neurosci Lett. 1997;223:197–200.

58. Marson L. Identification of central nervous system neurons that innervate the bladder body, bladder base, or external urethral sphincter of female rats: a transneuronal tracing study using pseudorabies virus. J Comp Neurol. 1997;389:584–602.

59. de Groat WC. Neural control of the urethra. Scand J Urol Nephrol. 2001;35(Suppl. 207):35–43.

60. De Groat WC, Ryall RW. Recurrent inhibition in sacral parasympathetic pathways to the bladder. J Physiol. 1968;196(3):579–91.

61. Athwal BS, Berkley KJ, Hussain I, et al. Brain responses to changes in bladder volume and urge to void in healthy men. Brain. 2001;124:369–77.

62. Griffiths D, Derbyshire S, Stenger A, et al. Brain control of normal and overactive bladder. J Urol. 2005;174:1862–7.

63. Kavia RB, Dasgupta R, Fowler CJ. Functional imaging and the central control of the bladder. J Comp Neurol. 2005;493:27–32.

64. Griffiths D, Tadic S. Bladder control, urgency, and urge incontinence: evidence from functional brain imaging. Neurourol Urodyn. 2008;27:466–74.

65. Willis WD, Al-Chaer ED, Quast MJ, et al. A visceral pain pathway in the dorsal column of the spinal cord. Proc Natl Acad Sci U S A. 1999;96:7675–9.

66. Chapple CR, Yamanishi T, Chess-Williams R. Muscarinic receptor subtypes and management of the overactive bladder. Urology. 2002;60:82–8.

67. de Groat WC, Yoshimura N. Pharmacology of the lower urinary tract. Annu Rev Pharmacol Toxicol. 2001;41:691–721.

68. Park JM, Bloom DA, McGuire EJ. The guarding reflex revisited. Br J Urol. 1997;80:940–5.

69. de Groat WC. Mechanisms underlying the recovery of lower urinary tract function following spinal cord injury. Paraplegia. 1995;33:493–505.

70. de Groat WC, Vizzard MA, Araki I, et al. Spinal interneurons and preganglionic neurons in sacral autonomic reflex pathways. Prog Brain Res. 1996;107:97–111.

71. de Groat WC. Integrative control of the lower urinary tract: preclinical perspective. Br J Pharmacol. 2006;147(Suppl. 2):S25–40.

72. Cockayne DA. Urinary bladder hyporeflexia and reduced pain-related behaviour in P2X3-deficient mice. Nature. 2000;407:1011–5.

73. Blok BF, Sturms LM, Holstege G. A PET study on cortical and subcortical control of pelvic floor musculature in women. J Comp Neurol. 1997;389:535–44.

74. Zhang H, Reitz A, Kollias S, et al. An fMRI study of the role of suprapontine brain structures in the voluntary voiding control induced by pelvic floor contraction. NeuroImage. 2005;24:174–80.

75. Seseke S, Baudewig J, Kallenberg K, et al. Voluntary pelvic floor muscle control—an fMRI study. NeuroImage. 2006;31:1399–407.

76. Kuhtz-Buschbeck JP, Van der Horst C, Wolff S, et al. Activation of the supplementary motor area (SMA) during voluntary pelvic floor muscle contractions-an fMRI study. NeuroImage. 2007;35:449–57.

77. Schrum A, Wolff S, Van der Horst C, et al. Motor cortical representation of the pelvic floor muscles. J Urol. 2011;186:185–90.

78. Holstege G, Griffiths D, De Wall H, et al. Anatomical and physiological observations on supraspinal control of bladder and urethral sphincter muscles in the cat. J Comp Neurol. 1986;250:449–61.

79. Griffiths DJ. The pontine micturition centres. Scand J Urol Nephrol. 2002;36(Suppl. 210): 21–6.

80. de Groat WC, Yoshimura N. Anatomy and physiology of the lower urinary tract. Handb Clin Neurol. 2015;130:61–108.

81. Kitta T, Mitsui T, Kanno Y, et al. Brain-bladder control network: the unsolved 21st century urological mystery. Int J Urol. 2015;22:342–8.

82. de Groat WC, Griffiths D, Yoshimura N. Neural control of the lower urinary tract. Compr Physiol. 2015;5:327–96.

83. Michels L, Blok BF, Gregorini F, et al. Supraspinal control of urine storage and micturition in men-an fMRI Study. Cereb Cortex. 2015;25:3369–80.

84. Sugaya K, Nishijima S, Miyazato M, et al. Inhibitory effect of the nucleus reticularis pontis oralis on the pontine micturition center and pontine urine storage center in decerebrate cats. Biomed Res. 2006;27:211–7.

85. Sakakibara R, Fowler CJ, Hattori T. Voiding and MRI analysis of the brain. Int Urogynecol J Pelvic Floor Dysfunct. 1999;10:192–9.

86. Blok BF, Holstege G. Two pontine micturition centers in the cat are not interconnected directly: implications for the central organization of micturition. J Comp Neurol. 1999;403:209–18.

87. Blok BF, Holstege G. The central nervous system control of micturition in cats and humans. Behav Brain Res. 1998;92:119–25.

88. de Groat WC. Nervous control of the urinary bladder of the cat. Brain Res. 1975;87:201–11.

89. Koyama Y, Ozaki H. KuruM. Interference between the pontine detrusor nucleus and the pontine urine-storage nucleus. An electromyographical study of the external urethral sphincter. Jpn J Physiol. 1966;16:291–303.

90. McGuire E, Morrissey S, Zhang S, et al. Control of reflex detrusor activity in normal and spinal injured nonhuman primates. J Urol. 1983;129:197–9.

91. de Groat WC. Inhibitory mechanisms in the sacral reflex pathways to the urinary bladder. In: Ryall RW, Kelly JS, editors. Iontophoresis and transmitter mechanisms in the mammalian central nervous system. Amsterdam: Elsevier; 1978.

92. de Groat WC, Booth AM, Milne RJ, et al. Parasympathetic preganglionic neurons in the sacral spinal cord. J Auton Nerv Syst. 1982;5:23–43.

93. de Groat WC. Central neural control of the lower urinary tract. Ciba Found Symp. 1990;151:27–44.

94. de Groat WC, Steers WD. Autonomic regulation of the urinary bladder and sex organs. In: Loewy AD, Spyer KM, editors. Central regulation of autonomic functions. 1st ed. Oxford University Press: Oxford; 1990.

95. de Groat WC. Neural control of urinary bladder and sexual organs. In: Bannister R, Mathias CJ, editors. Autonomic failure. 3rd ed. Oxford University Press: Oxford; 1992.

96. Nour S, Svarer C, Kristensen JK, et al. Cerebral activation during micturition in normal men. Brain. 2000;123:781–9.

97. Tai C, Jin T, Wang P, et al. Brain switch for reflex micturition control detected by fMRI in rats. J Neurophysiol. 2009;102:2719–30.

98. Matsuura S, Kakizaki H, Mitsui T, et al. Human brain region response to distention or cold stimulation of the bladder: a positron emission tomography study. J Urol. 2002;168:2035–9.

99. Blok B, Holstege G. Direct projections from the periaqueductal gray to the pontine micturition centre (M-region). An anterograde and retrograde tracing study in the cat. Neurosci Lett. 1994;166:93–6.
100. Shah AP, Mevcha A, Wilby D, et al. Continence and micturition: an anatomical basis. Clin Anat. 2014;27:1275–83.
101. Langworthy OR, Kolb LC. Demonstration of encephalic control of micturition by electrical stimulation. Bull Johns Hopkins Hosp. 1935:37–49.
102. Kabat H, Magoun HW, Ranson SW. Reaction of the bladder to stimulation of points in the forebrain and midbrain. J Comp Neurol. 1936;63:211–39.
103. Gjone R. Excitatory and inhibitory bladder responses to stimulation of 'limbic', diencephalic and mesencephalic structures in the cat. Acta Physiol Scand. 1966;66:91–102.
104. Koyama Y, Makuya A, Kuru M. Vesico-motor areas in the cat midbrain. Jpn J Physiol. 1962;12:63–80.
105. Skultety FM. Relation to periaqueductal gray matter to stomach and bladder motility. Neurology. 1959;9:190–8.
106. Numata A, Iwata T, Iuchi H, et al. Micturition suppressing region in the periaqueductal gray of the mesencephalon of the cat. Am J Phys. 2008;294:R1996–2000.
107. An X, Bandler R, Ongur D. Prefrontal cortical projections to longitudinal columns in the midbrain periaqueductal gray in macaque monkeys. J Comp Neurol. 1998;401:455–79.
108. Rosen SD, Paulesu E, Frith CD, et al. Central nervous pathways mediating angina pectoris. Lancet. 1994;344:147–50.
109. Weiller C, May A, Limmroth V, et al. Brain stem activation in spontaneous human migraine attacks. Nat Med. 1995;1:658–60.
110. Bandler R, Carrive P, Zhang SP. Integration of somatic and autonomic reactions within the midbrain periaqueductal gray: viscerotopic, somatotopic and functional organization. Prog Brain Res. 1991;87:269–305.
111. Holstege G, Bandler R, Saper CB. The emotional motor system. Prog Brain Res. 1996;107:3–6.
112. Van der Horst VG, Mouton LJ, Blok BF, et al. Distinct cell groups in the lumbosacral cord of the cat project to different areas in the periaqueductal gray. J Comp Neurol. 1996;376:361–85.
113. Taniguchi N, Miyata M, Yachiku S, et al. A study of micturition inducing sites in the periaqueductal gray of the mesencephalon. J Urol. 2002;168:1626–31.
114. Holstege G. How the emotional motor system controls the pelvic organs. Sex Med Rev. 2016;4:303–28.
115. Liu Z, Sakakibara R, Nakazawa K, et al. Micturition related neuronal firing in the periaqueductal gray area in cats. Neuroscience. 2004;126:1075–82.
116. Griffiths DJ, Fowler CJ. The micturition switch and its forebrain influences. Acta Physiol (Oxf). 2013;207:93–109.
117. Carmichael ST, Price JL. Connectional networks within the orbital and medial prefrontal cortex of macaque monkeys. J Comp Neurol. 1996;371:179–207.
118. Tang PC, Ruch TC. Localization of brain stem and diencephalic areas controlling the micturition reflex. J Comp Neurol. 1956;106:213–9.
119. Holstege G. Descending motor pathways and the spinal motor system: limbic and non-limbic components. Prog Brain Res. 1991;87:307–21.
120. Blok B, Willemsen T, Holstege G. A PET study of brain control of micturition in humans. Brain. 1997;120:111–21.
121. Blok BF, Holstege G. The central control of micturition and continence: implications for urology. Br J Urol Int. 1999;83(Suppl 2):1–6.
122. Sakakibara R, Nakazawa K, Shiba K, et al. Firing patterns of micturition-related neurons in the pontine storage centre in cats. Auton Neurosci. 2002;99:24–30.
123. Matsumoto G, Hisamitsu T, De Groat WC. Role of glutamate and NMDA receptors in the descending limb of the spinobulbospinal micturition reflex pathway of the rat. Neurosci Lett. 1995;183:58–61.

124. Valentino RJ, Chen S, Zhu Y, et al. Evidence for divergent projections to the brain noradrenergic system and the spinal parasympathetic system from Barrington's nucleus. Brain Res. 1996;732:1–15.
125. Betts CD, Kapoor R, Fowler CJ. Pontine pathology and voiding dysfunction. Br J Urol. 1992;70:100–2.
126. Sasaki M. Role of Barrington's nucleus in micturition. J Comp Neurol. 2005;493:21–6.
127. Swanson LW, Hartman BK. The central adrenergic system. An immunofluorescence study of the location of cell bodies and their efferent connections in the rat utilizing dopamine-beta-hydroxylase as a marker. J Comp Neurol. 1975;163:467–505.
128. Waterhouse BD, Devilbiss D, Fleischer D, et al. New perspectives on the functional organization and postsynaptic influences of the locus ceruleus efferent projection system. Adv Pharmacol. 1998;42:749–54.
129. Liu Y, Allen GV, Downie JW. Parabrachial nucleus influences the control of normal urinary bladder function and the response to bladder irritation in rats. Neuroscience. 2007;144:731–42.
130. Baez MA, Brink TS, Mason P. Roles for pain modulatory cells during micturition and continence. J Neurosci. 2005;25:384–94.
131. Kuipers R, Mouton LJ, Holstege G. Afferent projections to the pontine micturition center in the cat. J Comp Neurol. 2006;494:36–53.
132. Bradley WE, Teague CT. Cerebellar regulation of the micturition reflex. J Urol. 1969;101:396–99.
133. Nishizawa O, Sugaya K, Shimoda N. Pontine and spinal modulation of the micturition reflex. Scand J Urol Nephrol. Suppl 1995;175:15–9.
134. Ranson SW. Some functions of the hypothalamus: Harvey Lecture, December 17, 1936. Bull N Y Acad Med. 1937;13:241–71.
135. Enoch DM, Kerr FW. Hypothalamic vasopressor and vesicopressor pathways. II. Anatomic study of their course and connections. Arch Neurol. 1967;16:307–20.
136. Stuart DG, Portner RW, Adey WR, et al. Hypothalamic unit activity: visceral and somatic influences. Electroencephalogr Clin Neurophysiol. 1964;16:237–41.
137. Yoshimura N, Mizuta E, Yoshida O, et al. Therapeutic effects of dopamine D1/D2 receptor agonists on detrusor hyperreflexia in 1-methyl-4-phenyl-1,2,3,6-tetrahydropyridine—lesioned parkinsonian cynomolgus monkeys. J Pharmacol Exp Ther. 1998;286:228–33.
138. Seki S, Igawa Y, Kaidoh K, et al. Role of dopamine D1 and D2 receptors in the micturition reflex in conscious rats. Neurourol Urodyn. 2001;20:105–13.
139. Kitta T, Matsumoto M, Tanaka H, et al. GABAergic mechanism mediated via D receptors in the rat periaqueductal gray participates in the micturition reflex: an in vivo microdialysis study. Eur J Neurosci. 2008;27:3216–25.
140. Critchley HD, Wiens S, Rotshtein P, et al. Neural systems supporting interoceptive awareness. Nat Neurosci. 2004;7:189–95.
141. Salzman CD, Fusi S. Emotion, cognition, and mental state representation in amygdala and prefrontal cortex. Annu Rev Neurosci. 2010;33:173–202.
142. Schaefer DC, Cheskin LJ. Constipation in the elderly. Am Fam Physician. 1998;58:907–14.
143. Wald A, Hinds JP, Caruana BJ. Psychological and physiological characteristics of patients with severe idiopathic constipation. Gastroenterology. 1989;97:932–7.
144. Nehra V, Bruce BK, Rath-Harvey DM, et al. Psychological disorders in patients with evacuation disorders and constipation in a tertiary practice. Am J Gastroenterol. 2000;95:1755–8.
145. Dykes S, Smilgin-Humphreys S, Bass C. Chronic idiopathic constipation: a psychological enquiry. Eur J Gastroenterol Hepatol. 2001;13:39–44.
146. Partin JC, Hamill SK, Fischel JE, et al. Painful defecation and fecal soiling in children. Pediatrics. 1992;89:1007–9.
147. Rao SS, Sadeghi P, Beaty J, et al. Ambulatory 24-h colonic manometry in healthy humans. Am J Physiol Gastrointest Liver Physiol. 2001;280:G629–39.

148. Dinning PG, Zarate N, Szczesniak MM, et al. Bowel preparation affects the amplitude and spatiotemporal organization of colonic propagating sequences. Neurogastroenterol Motil. 2010;22:633–e176.
149. Bampton P, Dinning P, Kennedy M, Lubowski D, Cook I. Prolonged multi-point recording of colonic manometry in the unprepared human colon: providing insight into potentially relevant pressure wave parameters. Am J Gastroenterol. 2001;96:1838–48.
150. Bassotti G, Chistolini F, Nzepa F, Morelli A. Colonic propulsive impairment in intractable slow-transit constipation. Arch Surg. 2003;138:1302–4.
151. Palit S, Lunniss PJ, Scott SM. The physiology of human defecation. Dig Dis Sci. 2012;57(6):1445–64.
152. Bajwa A, Emmanuel A. The physiology of continence and evacuation. Best Pract Res Clin Gastroenterol. 2009;23:477–85.
153. Shafik A. Dilatation and closing anal reflexes. Description and clinical significance of new reflexes: preliminary report. Acta Anat (Basel). 1991;142:293–8.
154. Furness J, Callaghan B. Rivera L, et al. In: Lyte M, Cryan JF, editors. Microbial endocrinology: the microbiota-gut-brain axis in health and disease, advances in experimental medicine and biology. New York: Springer; 2014.
155. De Giorgio R, Lioce A, Barbara G, et al. Disordini della motilità gastrointestinale da alterazioni primitive del Sistema Nervoso Enterico. Neuro Gastroenterologia. 2003;3(4):51–62.
156. Bazzocchi G, Ellis J, Villanueva-Meyer J, et al. Effect of eating on colonic motility and transit in patients with functional diarrhea. Simultaneous scintigraphic and manometric evaluations. Gastroenterology. 1991;101:1298–306.
157. Bharucha A. Pelvic floor: anatomy and function. Neurogastroenterol Motil. 2006;18:507–19.
158. Altman J, Bayer SA. The development of the rat spinal cord. Adv Anat Embryol Cell Biol. 1984;85:1–14.
159. Vanner SJ, Greenwood-Van Meerveld B, Mawe GM, et al. Fundamentals of neurogastroenterology: basic science. Gastroenterology. 2016;150:1280–91.
160. Duthie HL, Gairns FW. Sensory nerve endings and sensation in the anal region of man. Br J Surg. 1960;47:585–95.
161. Goligher JC. The functional results after sphincter-saving resections of the rectum. Ann R Coll Surg Engl. 1951;8:421–38.
162. Sengupta JN, Gebhart GF. Characterization of mechanosensitive pelvic nerve afferent fibers innervating the colon of the rat. J Neurophysiol. 1994;71:2046–60.
163. Goligher JC, Hughes ES. Sensibility of the rectum and colon. Its role in the mechanism of anal continence. Lancet. 1951;1:543–7.
164. Burstein R, Cliffer KD, Giesler GJ. Direct somatosensory projections from the spinal cord to the hypothalamus and telencephalon. J Neurosci. 1987;7:4159–64.
165. Menetrey D, Basbaum AI. Spinal and trigeminal projections to the nucleus of the solitary tract: a possible substrate for somatovisceral and viscerovisceral reflex activation. J Comp Neurol. 1987;255:439–50.
166. Torvik A. Afferent connections to the sensory trigeminal nuclei, the nucleus of the solitary tract and adjacent structures; an experimental study in the rat. J Comp Neurol. 1956;106:51–141.
167. Sato A, Schmidt RF. Somatosympathetic reflexes: afferent fibers, central pathways, discharge characteristics. Physiol Rev. 1973;53:916–47.
168. Valentino RJ, Miselis RR, Pavcovich LA. Pontine regulation of pelvic viscera: pharmacological target for pelvic visceral dysfunction. Trends Pharmacol Sci. 1999;20:253–60.
169. Kiddoo DA, Valentino RJ, Zderic S, et al. Impact of state of arousal and stress neuropeptides on urodynamic function in freely moving rats. Am J Physiol Regul Integr Comp Physiol. 2006;290:R1697–706.

170. Suzuki T, Sugiyama Y, Yates BJ. Integrative responses of neurons in parabrachial nuclei to a nauseogenic gastrointestinal stimulus and vestibular stimulation in vertical planes. Am J Physiol Regul Integr Comp Physiol. 2012;302:R965–75.
171. Tache Y, Bonaz B. Corticotropin-releasing factor receptors and stress-related alterations of gut motor function. J Clin Invest. 2007;117:33–40.
172. Rouzade-Dominguez ML, Pernar L, Beck S, et al. Convergent responses of Barrington's nucleus neurons to pelvic visceral stimuli in the rat: a juxtacellular labelling study. Eur J Neurosci. 2003;18:3325–34.
173. Kalia M, Sullivan JM. Brainstem projections of sensory and motor components of the vagus nerve in the rat. J Comp Neurol. 1982;211:248–64.
174. Rogers J. Testing for and the role of anal and rectal sensation. Bailliere's Clin Gastroenterol. 1992;6:179–91.
175. Brookes SJ, Dinning PG, Gladman MA. Neuroanatomy and physiology of colorectal function and defaecation: from basic science to human clinical studies. Neurogastroenterol Motil. 2009;21:9–19.
176. Lomax AE, Sharkey KA, Furness JB. The participation of the sympathetic innervation of the gastrointestinal tract in disease states. Neurogastroenterol Motil. 2010;22:7–18.
177. Janig W, McLachlan EM. Organization of lumbar spinal outflow to distal colon and pelvic organs. Physiol Rev. 1987;67:1332–404.
178. Simmons MA. The complexity and diversity of synaptic transmission in the prevertebral sympathetic ganglia. Prog Neurobiol. 1985;24:43–93.
179. Sakakibara R, Kishi M, Ogawa E, et al. Bladder, bowel, and sexual dysfunction in Parkinson's disease. Parkinson's Dis. 2011;2011:924605.

2

Donatella Giraudo and Francesco Verderosa

2.1 The Somatic Component

Somatic, parasympathetic and sympathetic components innervate the organs contained in the pelvis. The clinical evaluation of the perineum sensitivity must pay particular attention to the fact that adjacent areas of skin surface (adjacent dermatomes such as L1–L2 and S2–S3) refer to metamers which are well distant at a spinal cord level: during development, in fact, the rotation of the lower limb causes this apparently unordered distribution [1].

The sensitivity evaluation of the perineal area is performed on the supine patient with his/her hip and knee bent, in order to explore the various areas which will be stimulated, usually with a cotton stick, to evaluate the exteroceptive tactile and pain sensibility, including visually.

The "touch" of the cotton stick aims to explore the urogenital and the anal triangle, which are both innervated by the pudendal nerve [2–5], with some thoracolumbar nerves overlapping with it in this area.

The anterior branches of the spinal nerves from T12 to L4 form the lumbar plexus, which has close relations with the posterior abdominal wall, running along the psoas muscle; the sympathetic afferents run in the upper hypogastric plexus, while the parasympathetic ones in the inferior hypogastric plexus.

Anterior cutaneous branches from T7 to T12 provide the somatic innervation of the abdominal wall; in particular, the area innervated by the iliohypogastric

D. Giraudo (✉)
Urology Department, San Raffaele Turro Hospital, Milan, Italy
e-mail: giraudo.donatella@hsr.it

F. Verderosa
Spinal Unit and Intensive Rehabilitation Medicine A.U.S.L. Piacenza,
Emilia Romagna Region, Italy
e-mail: f.verderosa@ausl.pc.it

© Springer Nature Switzerland AG 2020
G. Lamberti et al. (eds.), *Suprapontine Lesions and Neurogenic Pelvic Dysfunctions*, Urodynamics, Neurourology and Pelvic Floor Dysfunctions,
https://doi.org/10.1007/978-3-030-29775-6_2

nerve includes the superior lateral skin portion of the buttock and comes up to the suprapubic skin.

The ilioinguinal nerve and the genital branch of the genitofemoral nerve contribute to the sensory innervation of the skin of the labia majora, scrotum and pubis (Figs. 2.1 and 2.2).

The sacral plexus is formed by the roots L4–S4, emerges from the sacral foramen and moves sideways in close contact with the piriformis muscle, innervated by the first and second sacral nerves.

The inferior gluteal nerve (posterior branches of L4, L5 and S1) innervates the gluteus maximus muscle, passing below the piriformis muscle; the femoral cutaneous provides innervation to the anterolateral part of the perineum [6, 7].

There are some controversies about the constitution of the pudendal nerve trunk: it is usually described as originating from S2, S3 and S4; there are some observations which hypothesise a contribution also of the S1 root [8–10].

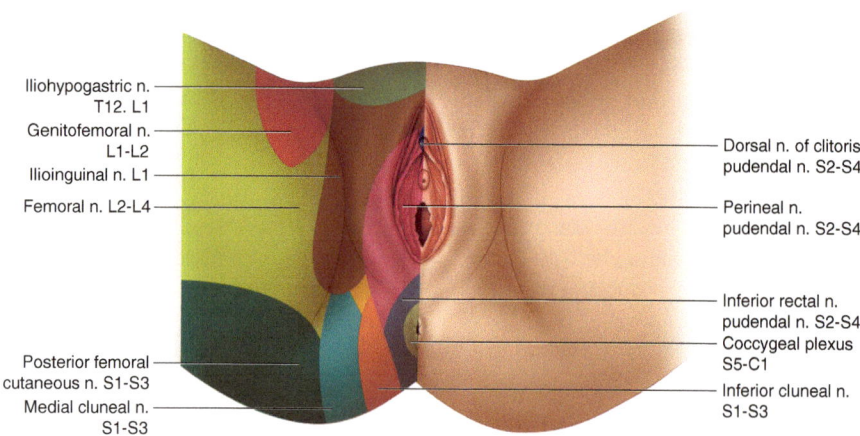

Fig. 2.1 Sensory innervation in the female perineum

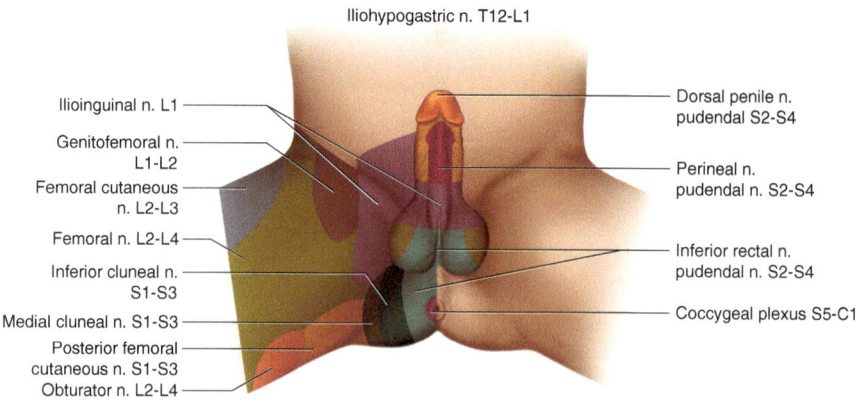

Fig. 2.2 Sensory innervation of the male perineum

Running between the piriformis muscle and the coccygeal muscle, it enters the perineum through the small ischial foramen, and runs in the Alcock's canal to then divide into its terminal branches. The pudendal nerve guarantees the sensitivity of the anterior and posterior perineum, conveying within itself afferent but also efferent somatic fibres, sympathetic and parasympathetic efferent fibres and visceral afferent fibres [2–5, 11, 12].

The dorsal nerve of the clitoris (in the female) and the dorsal penile nerve (in the male) run along the ischiopubic ramus and provide skin innervation to the clitoris or the penis; a second branch, the inferior rectal nerve, after having run through the Alcock's canal reaches the perianal area, ensuring motor and sensory somatic innervation to the external anal sphincter, the anal canal and the adjacent cutaneous area [13–15]. The last branch, the perineal nerve, provides innervation of the cutaneous area corresponding to the perineal body; its deep component supplies the transverse muscles of the perineum, the bulbospongiosus muscle, the ischiocavernosus muscle and part of the external anal sphincter.

The coccygeal plexus is formed by a small branch descending from the IV sacral root, the V sacral root and the ventral coccygeal branch. The V sacral root exits the sacral hiatus, and crosses the coccygeal muscle to reach the perineum. The levator ani muscles and the coccygeal muscle, together with the sacrococcygeal articulation and the skin over the anococcygeal raphe, are innervated by the coccygeal plexus.

The sensory innervation of the anus and rectum ensures two functions: the rectal "sampling" and the detection of the degree of distension of the rectal walls in order to trigger the recto-anal inhibitory reflex (RAIR) for beginning the defecation or, on the contrary, the voluntary contraction of the muscle-sphincter complex to postpone it and the anal sensitivity [16, 17].

In the anorectal area, the afferent nerve impulses are conveyed by the pudendal nerve [18] by both myelinated and non-myelinated fibres [19].

2.2 The Sympathetic and Parasympathetic Components

The greater splanchnic nerve (from the sympathetic thoracolumbar fibres T5 to T9) connects with the celiac plexus and innervates the small intestine and the colon. The fibres from T10 and T11 form the minor splanchnic nerve which equally innervates, through the upper mesenteric plexus, the small intestine and the colon; the last splanchnic nerves originate from T12 and send fibres to the renal and ovarian plexuses [14, 20].

The lumbar splanchnic nerves, through the inferior mesenteric plexus, in part innervate the colon and through the rectal upper plexus the rectum, the anal canal and the internal anal sphincter; in the caudal area, it takes the name of superior hypogastric plexus (exclusively sympathetic plexus), which innervates the sigmoid, ureters and uterus. Each hypogastric nerve receives a component from the sacral splanchnic nerves and forms the pelvic plexus (inferior hypogastric plexus) with a sympathetic and parasympathetic double component, which innervates the bladder (bladder plexus), the uterus and vagina (uterovaginal plexus) and the rectum (rectal plexus).

The parasympathetic system has a sacral protrusion with fibres that originate from the cranial nerves with some components of the sacral spinal nerves. In contrast to the sympathetic neurons, preganglionic fibres contract synapses with the postganglionic fibres in the vicinity of the target organs. The abdominal-pelvic area is innervated mainly by the vagus nerve; the vagal fibres join sympathetic fibres in the upper and lower mesenteric and celiac plexuses and contract synapses with the postganglionic fibres in the enteric ganglia (in the Meissner and Auerbach plexuses) to innervate the small intestine, colon, kidneys and ureters. The sacral parasympathetic fibres (anterior branches of S2, S3 and S4) innervate the digestive tract and the urogenital organs through the pelvic plexus.

2.2.1 Clinical Evaluation of Reflexes

2.2.1.1 Surface or Exteroceptive Reflexes (Polysynaptic Reflexes)

The evaluation of reflexes allows the possibility of identifying the level of injury in the CNS during a general neurological examination. Put simply, all reflexes represent a sensorimotor arc with a single link between the afferent branch and the efferent one (monosynaptic reflex) or with one or more interposed neurons (polysynaptic reflex). They can be controlled by inhibitory and/or excitatory influences that reach the spinal level, originating from different areas of the CNS, which are therefore able, in the presence of any disease, to modify the reflex response. Superficial or exteroceptive reflexes are mediated by a polysynaptic arch, therefore substantially different from monosynaptic proprioceptive reflexes, since their processing takes place thanks to the intervention of interneurons also at a supraspinal level; the receptors consist of mechanoreceptors and nociceptors of the skin and mucosa, the afferent pathway of T cells with myelinated axons and the efferent pathway from the alpha motor neurons. In the case of exteroceptive reflexes, the stimulus and the response to the stimulus are shown in different organs or apparatuses, and different peripheral nerves or nerve roots represent the afferent pathway and the efferent pathway of the reflex; usually triggered by stimulating the skin with a "rubbing" movement (usually the stimulation is carried out with a rigid and rounded object, in this case, a wooden stick), these are evaluated as "present" or "absent", considering that marked-side asymmetries must be considered as pathological.

The repeated attempt to trigger the reflex makes the response less evident and exhaustible.

Their abolition may be secondary to a lesion of the afferent nerves or the second motor neuron efferent and of all cases of interruption between the brain and spinal cord [21].

2.2.2 Abdominal Reflexes

Originally described by Rosenbach [22], it is recommended that they should be triggered initially by using the Wartenberg "pinwheel" [23]. Currently, it is suggested to cause the contraction of the abdominal muscles by stimulating the peri-umbilical skin with a blunt tip with a movement in the latero-medial direction towards the navel, performed bilaterally in the four abdominal quadrants, above and below the navel [24], with the patient in a supine position, relaxed, looking for reflexes at the end of an exhalation; the afferent nerve impulses are conveyed by the intercostal, ilioinguinal and iliohypogastric nerves [25].

The contraction generally determines the "displacement" of the navel itself towards the stimulated quadrant; it is, therefore, possible to trigger superior or epigastric reflexes (spinal segments T7–T9), medium reflexes (T9–T11) and inferior reflexes (T11–T12, overlapping with L1) [26].

They can be very lively in case of an anxious state or of a long-standing corticospinal lesion [27] and bilaterally absent in 15% of the population, in the elderly person, in the obese person and in the multipara. They are absent on one side in case of interruption of the reflex arc (shingles, abdominal surgery outcome, lesions of the second motor neuron), as well as in the case of an ipsi- or contralateral lesion of the cranial-spinal tract at the examined level. They can therefore assist in the diagnosis of thoracic spinal cord injuries [27].

An "inverse" response may rarely be triggered with a contraction of the contralateral muscles related to stimulation; they may be precociously absent in case of multiple sclerosis [28], a sign described by Ernst Adolf Gustav Gottfried von Strümpell in 1896.

They can be triggered instead in case of amyotrophic lateral sclerosis and of myasthenia gravis [26].

2.2.2.1 "Deep" Abdominal Reflexes

"Deep" abdominal reflexes have been described, triggered not by stimulating the skin of the abdomen, but by stretching the musculature itself, activating it with the hammer or Wartenberg pinwheel on the abdominal wall [29]. The absence of superficial ones in the presence of accentuated deep reflexes (dissociation between "deep" and "superficial" abdominal reflexes [30]) would suggest a bilateral lesion of the pyramidal tract above the T6 [31, 32].

2.2.3 The Cremasteric Reflex (in the Male)

Described by Monrad-Krohn and Kornfeldt in 1925, it is triggered by stimulating the afferent fibres of the ilioinguinal nerve in the medial area of the thigh and with the efferent motor response of the genital branch of the genitofemoral nerve [33]; the cremasteric muscle determines the elevation of the testis on the same side where the stimulation occurred.

Present after 2 years of age, the reflex cannot always be triggered even under normal conditions; it assesses the L1–L2 segment: it may be important in the diagnosis of lesions at the lumbar plexus, in diabetic neuropathy, lymphomas, autoimmune diseases and rarely Lyme disease or polyarteritis nodosa.

It can be absent in elderly persons or in the outcome of abdominal surgery for hernia or hydrocele or in lesions of the L1–L2 cranial contralateral pyramidal tract or L1–L2 spinal lesions [34–36].

The cremasteric reflex is a somatic motor reflex; it has also been described as the "dartos reflex" [33] or "scrotal reflex", an autonomic reflex, but clinically similar to the cremasteric reflex since the afferent and efferent arcs of the reflexes differ only in the "dartos reflex for the sympathetic component" [37].

The dartos muscle is a cutaneous smooth muscle which adheres tightly to the deep layer of the scrotal bag skin, of which it is a tunica. Similarly to the cremasteric muscle, it receives fibres from the genitofemoral nerve, in particular also from a contingent of fibres of the sympathetic nervous system, which originate in the thoracolumbar cord (T12-L1-L2). This component is responsible for the "corrugation" of the scrotal skin, which manifests itself with a slightly higher latency than the testicular elevation [35, 37].

Triggering both reflexes thus confirms the integrity of the cord metamers T12 and L1 and of the afferent and efferent arcs; the presence of the "dartos reflex" also demonstrates the integrity of the autonomic innervation of the scrotum [38].

2.2.4   The Anocutaneous Reflex, Anal Wink, Anal Reflex, Perineal Reflex

Originally described by Rossolimo, the anocutaneous reflex is evidenced by the contraction of the external anal sphincter (EAS) (efferent fibres from S2-S3-S4), stimulated by cutaneous afferents of the pudendal nerve [39]. Its presence, according to authors, inserted in an anticipatory motor pattern with the increase of the intra-abdominal pressure when coughing [40], is indicative for the integrity of the S4 level; easily exhaustible, it is absent in geriatric age and, often, in cord lesions (like other polysynaptic superficial reflexes), of cauda equina and in lesions of the sacral roots.

In suprasegmental lesions of the central nervous system, the reflex did not differ from healthy subjects; however, it could be more pronounced and with a duration of a few seconds [41].

The superficial anal reflex or "anal wink" consists of the contraction of the subcutaneous portion [42, 43] of the EAS in response to stimulation of the skin or mucosa in the perianal area. After a short latency, the contraction first appears homolaterally to stimulation and subsequently contralaterally [44]. The reflex is mediated by the lower haemorrhoidal nerve (S3-S5) and is probably controlled by encephalic centres [45, 46].

The evaluation of the superficial anal reflex is particularly critical for the diagnosis of cauda equina or conus medullaris syndrome: the simultaneous absence and presence of the voluntary contraction of the EAS with the presence of the reflex and tone of the EAS are indicative of a suprasacral lesion.

The superficial anal reflex and the bulbocavernosus reflex are somatic motor reflexes while the internal anal reflex and the scrotal reflexes are autonomic reflexes [47].

The internal anal reflex is elicited when a gloved finger reaches the internal anal sphincter; if the reflex is altered (absence of the reflex contraction of the internal anal sphincter), there is a reduced sphincter tone and a non-immediate closure after defecation [41, 43].

2.2.5 Clitoral-Anal Reflex/Bulbocavernosus Reflex

The bulbocavernosus (or clitoral-anal reflex in the woman) or bulbospongiosus reflex or "Osinski reflex" [48] is a polysynaptic reflex which determines the contraction of the pelvic floor muscles at the compression of the glans or clitoris [49]. Initially described as a reflex capable of invoking the contraction of the bulbocavernosus and ischiocavernosus muscles [50], it was subsequently "modified" giving more emphasis on the contraction of the EAS [51], accessible to the examiner's view or to the touch.

The compression of the glans penis (or clitoris) is carried out with delicate but firm compressions at intervals of 4–5 s [50, 52–55]; the stimulation uses the afference of the root S2 and the contraction of the bulbocavernosus muscle and the EAS are provided by the S4 and S5 roots.

The reflex is essential for the evaluation of the conus medullaris and the sacral cord metamers; in case of lesion of the cauda equina, it can be absent [56] and generally triggered in case of injury of the superior motor neuron [57].

The conus medullaris and the first lumbar vertebra are usually at the same level: a lesion of the 11th or 12th thoracic vertebra can cause suprasacral lesions of the cord, while a fracture of the first lumbar vertebra may involve sacral metamers.

The simultaneous presence of the superficial anal reflex and the bulbocavernosus (or clitoral-anal) reflex allows hypothesising a normal condition of the second, third and fourth sacral metamers, while its absence a lesion of the second motoneuron or of the corresponding sacral myelomeres; physiologically it may not be present in 20% of women without any neurological disease.

2.2.6 Guarding Reflex

Several authors have studied the increase in pressure which can be measured at the urethral level while coughing or the Valsalva manoeuvre [58, 59]; in addition to the response not equally distributed throughout the urethra (more significant at the distal level), an anticipation of the increase in urethral pressure of about 250 ms compared with the bladder one was also observed. The anticipated reflex activation of the pelvic floor, also demonstrated by ultrasound [60], is controlled by the CNS [61–63]. Clinically it may be triggered by asking the person being examined to cough and observing the "holding" movement of the pelvic floor (more easily detectable in a woman) or, in doubtful cases, by evaluating the palpation of PFM.

There is a response in people with a complete cord lesion above the lumbar level [62], and it is almost always absent in postpartum (although in this last case—as in all situations characterised by stress urinary incontinence [63, 64]—probably myofascial factors, dependant on the thoracolumbar fascia and the transverse muscle of the abdomen, play an essential role).

The reflex may be found in incomplete spinal cord injuries and suprapontine lesions [65].

The lack of "guarding reflex" supraspinal control in suprasacral spinal cord lesions is at the basis of the vesico-sphincter dyssynergia which occurs in this clinical situation [66], and its alteration could be involved in a detrusor overactivity not correlated with clear neurological pictures [67].

2.3 Reflex Alterations and Clinical Pictures

Reflexes are altered in case of pathological situations which compromise the recruitment of the muscles activated by the efferent arc, such as in the case of large scar tissues or the degeneration of muscle fibres observed at the IAS in systemic sclerosis or of the EAS in ALS [68, 69].

In the case of peripheral neuropathies, reflex responses can be precociously compromised, often not corresponding to the recruitment deficit (often minimal), due to the early and prevailing involvement of the afferent component of the reflex itself. In radiculopathies, reflexes can often be normal due to the joint participation of several roots in producing the reflected arc itself; the extensive damage of several roots, however, determines the disappearance of the affected reflexes (cauda equina syndrome) in association with a sensitivity deficit and reduced muscle recruitment.

Superficial reflexes are absent in case of injury of the spinal metamer involved and often absent or normal in case of injury above the metamer itself (epicone syndrome caused by a spinal cord injury to the T11–T12 vertebra). In particular, in case of lesion of the corticospinal tract, it is possible to observe their absence but, in particular as concerns abdominal reflexes, it is essential to correlate the datum to the remaining clinical picture: advanced age, abdominal scars, obesity and multiparity are often associated with their absence.

No significant changes in surface reflexes are observed in cases of cerebellar lesions or those of basal ganglia. In the case of a unilateral encephalic lesion, there is a pattern characterised by the accentuation of proprioceptive reflexes, together with the reduction of superficial reflexes, contralateral to the lesion; bilateral lesions will determine bilaterally similar patterns [70, 71].

References

1. Tarulli AW. Disorders of the cauda equina. Continuum (Minneap Minn). 2015;21:146–58.
2. Robert R, Labat JJ, Riant T, et al. Somatic perineal pain other than pudendal neuralgia. Neurochirurgie. 2009;55(4–5):470–4.
3. Bensignor-Le Henaff M, Labat JJ, Robert T, et al. Perineal pain and lesions of the internal pudendal nerves. Cah Anesthesiol. 1993;41(2):111–4.
4. Bensignor-Le Henaff M, Labat JJ, Robert R, Lajat Y, et al. Perineal pain and involvement of the internal pudendal nerves. Agressologie. 1991;32:277–9.

5. Bouchet A, Cuilleret J. Anatomie topographique descriptive et fonctionnelle, tome 3b, Le membre inferieur. 3e éd ed. Paris: Simep/Masson; 1995.
6. Kamina P. Précis d'anatomie clinique, tome I. 1re éd ed. Paris: Maloine; 2002.
7. Rouvière H, Delmas A, Delmas V. Anatomie humaine descriptive, topographique et fonctionnelle, tome 3, Membres. 15e éd ed. Paris: Masson; 2002.
8. Marani E, Pijl MEJ, Kraan MC, et al. Interconnection of the upper ventral rami of the human sacral plexus: a reappraisal for dorsal rhizotomy in neurostimulation operations. Neurourol Urodyn. 1993;12:585–98.
9. Jünemann K, Lue TF, Schmidt RA, et al. Clinical significance of sacral and pudendal nerve anatomy. J Urol. 1988;139:74.
10. Gil-Vernet S. Innervation somatique et végétative des organes génito-urinaires. Acta Urol Belg. 1964;32:265–93.
11. Labat JJ, Robert R, Bensignor M, et al. Les névralgies du nerf pudendal (honteux interne). Considérations anatomocliniques et perspectives thérapeutiques. J Urol (Paris). 1990;96:239–44.
12. Vodušek DB, Light JK. The motor nerve supply of the external urethral sphincter muscles. Neurourol Urodyn. 1983;2:193–200.
13. Vodušek DB. Anatomy and neurocontrol of the pelvic floor. Digestion. 2004;69(2):87–92.
14. Mohammadali M, Sharma A, Mirza N, et al. Neuroanatomy of the female abdominopelvic region: a review with application to pelvic pain syndromes. Clin Anat. 2013;26:66–76.
15. Hoffman B, Schorge J, Schaffer J, et al. Williams gynecology. 2nd ed. New York: McGraw Hill Professional; 2012.
16. Benezech A, Bouvier M, Vitton V. Faecal incontinence: current knowledges and perspectives. World J Gastrointest Pathophysiol. 2016;7:59–71.
17. Fry P, Chess-Williams R, Hashitani H, et al. Cell biology. In: Abrams P, Cardozo L, Wagg A, Wein A, editors. Incontinence: 6th International Consultation on Incontinence, Tokyo, September 2016, vol. 1. 6th ed. Bristol (UK): International Continence Society (ICS) and International Consultation on Urological Diseases (ICUD); 2017.
18. Remes-Troche JM, Rao SS. Neurophysiological testing in anorectal disorders. Exp Rev Gastroenterol Hepatol. 2008;2:323–35.
19. Rao SS. Pathophysiology of adult fecal incontinence. Gastroenterology. 2004;126:S14–22.
20. Roberts M. Clinical neuroanatomy of the abdomen and pelvis: implications for surgical treatment of prolapse. Clin Obstet Gynecol. 2005;48(3):627–38.
21. Schwartzman RJ. Differential diagnosis in Neurology. Amsterdam: I.O.S. Press; 2006.
22. Rosenbach O. Ein Beitrag zur Symptomatologie cerebraler Hemiplegieen. Arch Psychiatr Nervenkr. 1876;6:845–51.
23. Wartenberg R. A pinwheel for neurologic examination. JAMA. 1937;109:1294.
24. Monrad-Krohn GH. Technique clinique d'examen complet du systeme nerveux. Paris: Librairie E. le Francois; 1925.
25. Mumenthaler M. Neurologic differential diagnosis. New York: Thieme Stratton; 1985.
26. Dick JPR. The deep tendon and the abdominal reflexes. J Neurol Neurosurg Psychiatry. 2003;74:150–3.
27. Walton JN. Brain's diseases of the nervous system. 7th ed. Oxford: Oxford University Press; 1969.
28. McAlpine D, Lumsden CE, Acheson ED. Multiple sclerosis, a reappraisal. London: Livingstone; 1965.
29. Wartenberg R. The examination of reflexes, a simplification. Chicago: The Year book publishers; 1945.
30. Lehoczky T, Fodors T. Clinical significance of the dissociation of abdominal reflexes. Neurology. 1953;3:453–9.
31. Monrad-Krohn GH. The clinical examination of the nervous system. 3rd ed. London: HK Lewis; 1926.
32. Hargrove G, Bors E. The suprapubic abdominal tap reflex: a useful method to assess the function of the sacral reflex arcs. J Urol. 1972;107:243–4.

33. Yilmaz U, Yang CC, Berger RE. Dartos reflex: a sympathetically mediated scrotal reflex. Muscle Nerve. 2006;33(3):363–8.
34. Bingol-Kologlu M, Demirci M, Buyukpamukcu N, et al. Cremasteric reflexes of boys with descended, retractile, or undescended testes: an electrophysiological evaluation. J Pediatr Surg. 1999;34:430–4.
35. Nagy JI, Senba E. Neural relations of cremaster motoneurons, spinal cord systems and the genitofemoral nerve in the rat. Brain Res Bull. 1985;15:609–27.
36. Haerer A. The superficial cutaneous reflexes. In: Haerer A, editor. De Jong's the neurologic examination. London: Lippincott; 1992.
37. Yang CC, Bradley WE. Somatic innervation of the human bulbocavernosus muscle. Clin Neurophysiol. 1999;110:412–8.
38. Schwarz GM, Hirtler L. The cremasteric reflex and its muscle—a paragon of ongoing scientific discussion: a systematic review. Clin Anat. 2017;30(4):498–507.
39. Rossolimo G. Der Analreflex, seine physiologie und pathologie. Neurologisches Centralblatt. 1891;4:257–9.
40. Cavallari P, Bolzoni F, Esposti R, et al. Cough-anal reflex may be the expression of a pre-programmed postural action. Front Hum Neurosci. 2017;11:475.
41. Pedersen E. Human anal reflexes. In: Henry MM, Swash M, editors. Coloproctology and the pelvic floor. London: Butterworths; 1985. p. 104–11.
42. Steele S, Hull T, Read T, Saclarides T, Senagore A, Whitlow C, editors. The ASCRS textbook of colon and rectal surgery. 3rd ed. Oakbrook Terrace, IL: ASCRS; 2016.
43. Deep Tendon Reflexes. http://stanfordmedicine25.stanford.edu/the25/tendon.html. Accessed 29 Jun 2019.
44. Swash M, Mathers S. Sphincter disorders and the nervous system. In: Aminoff M, editor. Neurology and general medicine. New York, NY: Churchill-Livingstone; 1989.
45. Chan CL, Ponsford S, Swash M. The anal reflex elicited by cough and sniff: validation of a neglected clinical sign. J Neurol Neurosurg Psychiatry. 2004;75(10):1449–51.
46. Frenckner B. Function of the anal sphincters in spinal man. Gut. 1975;16:482–9.
47. Campbell WW. DeJong's the neurologic examination. Philadelphia, PA: Lippincott Williams & Wilkins; 2013.
48. Chancellor M, Blaivas J. Practical neurourology: genitourinary complications in neurologic disease. Oxford: Butterworth-Heinemann; 1985.
49. Rattner W, Gerlaugh R, Murphy J, et al. The bulbocavernosus reflex: electromyographic study of normal patients. J Urol. 1958;80(2):140–1.
50. Rushton DN. Neuro-urological history and examination. In: Handbook of neuro-urology. New York, Basel, Hong Kong: Marcel Dekker; 1994.
51. Bors E, Blinn KA. Bulbocavernosus reflex. J Urol. 1959;82(1):128–30.
52. Wester C, FitzGerald MP, Brubaker L, et al. Validation of the clinical bulbocavernosus reflex. Neurourol Urodyn. 2003;22(6):589–91.
53. Blaivas JG, Chancellor MB. Neuro-urologic examination. In: Chancellor MB, Blaivas JG, editors. Practical neuro-urology. Genitourinary complications in neurologic disease. Boston, Oxford: Butterworth-Heinemann; 1995.
54. Khullar V, Cardozo L. History and examination. In: Cardozo L, Staskin D, editors. Textbook of female urology and urogynaecology. London: ISIS Medical Media; 2001.
55. Stanton SL. History and examination. In: Stanton SL, Monga AK, editors. Clinical urogynaecology. 2nd ed. London: Churchill Livingstone; 2000.
56. Blaivas JG, Zayed AA, Labib KB. The bulbocavernosus reflex in urology: a prospective study of 299 patients. J Urol. 1981;126:197–9.
57. Bobbitt JM, Lapides J. Diagnostic value of bulbocavernosus reflex. J Am Med Assoc. 1956;162(10):971–2.
58. Constantinou CE, Govan DE. Spatial distribution and timing of transmitted and reflexly generated urethral pressures in healthy women. J Urol. 1982;127(5):964–9.
59. Craggs MD, Balasubramaniam AV, Chung EA, et al. Aberrant reflexes and function of the pelvic organs following spinal cord injury in man. Auton Neurosci. 2006;126:355–70.

60. Dietz HP, Erdmann M, Shek KL. Reflex contraction of the levator ani and external peri-neal muscles in women symptomatic for pelvic floor disorders. Ultrasound Obstet Gynecol. 2012;40:215–8.
61. Enck P, Vodusek DB. Electromyography of pelvic floor muscles. J Eletromyogr Kinesiol. 2006;16:568–77.
62. Amarenco G, Ismael S, Lagauche D, et al. Cough anal reflex: strict relationship between intra-vesical pressure and pelvic floor muscle electromyographic activity during cough. Urodynamic and electrophysiological study. J Urol. 2005;173:149–52.
63. Deffieux X, Raibaut P, Rene-Corail P, et al. External anal sphincter contraction during cough: not a simple spinal reflex. Neurourol Urodyn. 2006;25:782–7.
64. Chancellor MB, Perkin H, Yoshimura N. Recent advances in the neurophysiology of stress urinary incontinence. Scand J Urol Nephrol. 2005;39:21–4.
65. Siroky MB, Krane RJ. Neurologic aspects of detrusor-sphincter dyssynergia, with reference to the guarding reflex. J Urol. 1982;127:953–7.
66. Rudy DC, Awad SA, Downie JW. External sphincter dyssynergia: an abnormal continence reflex. J Urol. 1988;140:105–10.
67. Park JM, Bloom DA, McGuire EJ. The guarding reflex revisited. Br J Urol. 1997;80(6):940–5.
68. Fynne L, Luft F, Gregersen H, et al. Distensibility of the anal canal in patients with systemic sclerosis: a study with the functional lumen imaging probe. Color Dis. 2013;15(1):e40–7.
69. Mannen T, Iwata M, Toyokura Y, et al. The Onuf's nucleus and the external anal sphincter muscles in amyotrophic lateral sclerosis and Shy-Drager syndrome. Acta Neuropathol. 1982;58:255–60.
70. DeJong RN. The neurologic examination. 4th ed. New York: Paul B. Hoeber; 1958.
71. Monrad-Krohn GH, Refsum S. The clinical examination of the nervous system. 12th ed. London: H.K. Lewis; 1964.

Investigation of the Central Nervous System in Neurogenic Pelvic Dysfunctions by Imaging

3

Achim Herms and Alida M. R. Di Gangi Herms

3.1 Introduction

Several suprapontine structures contribute to the functional control of the pelvic organs, of micturition, defecation, continence and sexual function. They are coordinated in complex networks that are able to adapt themselves to altered conditions.

Damage to those suprapontine structures provokes basically a limited number of different clinical conditions: retention, incontinence, urgency and sexual dysfunction.

On the other hand, these clinical conditions themselves may cause functional modifications of the suprapontine structures as long as at least some connectivity with the cerebral structures is upheld. Psychological distress may contribute to the onset of an overactive bladder [1].

It is unclear to which point neurogenic pelvic dysfunctions are direct consequences of the damage of a defined structure or whether they are the sum of interdependent phenomena.

Therefore, it could be hypothesized that the recovery of neurogenic pelvic dysfunctions depends not only on the healing process of the CNS itself, but also on the way the involved areas as well as the pelvic organs will react and interact.

A. Herms (✉)
Department of Urology, General Hospital Bressanone, Azienda Sanitaria dell'Alto Adige, Bressanone, Italy
e-mail: Achim.herms@sabes.it

A. M. R. D. G. Herms
Department of Psychology, General Hospital Bressanone, Azienda Sanitaria dell'Alto Adige, Bressanone, Italy
e-mail: alida.digangi@sabes.it

© Springer Nature Switzerland AG 2020
G. Lamberti et al. (eds.), *Suprapontine Lesions and Neurogenic Pelvic Dysfunctions*, Urodynamics, Neurourology and Pelvic Floor Dysfunctions, https://doi.org/10.1007/978-3-030-29775-6_3

The conventional MRI and CT scan-based diagnosis of the damage of a cerebral area may well give hints about a possible subsequent neurogenic pelvic dysfunction—but only up to a certain degree.

The last two decades have seen a dramatic evolution of new techniques to investigate brain function. Actually, they may still have a limited clinical applicability in daily activity and only a limited number of algorithms of their use exist. Nevertheless, in the same way that the introduction of the PSA has boosted the development of the therapy of prostate cancer, it is to be expected that more sophisticated diagnostics will lead to a more efficient and punctual, a more tolerable and cheaper management of patients with neurogenic pelvic dysfunctions.

The goal of this chapter is to provide an introduction to the techniques of investigation of the suprapontine structures and to the evolution of the knowledge they have created.

3.2   What Do We Know About Methodology?

Conventional CT and MRI scans may correlate the site of cerebral lesions with the probability of the presence of a certain type of pelvic dysfunctions [2]. Functional brain imaging, instead, provides information about the activation of brain areas in relation to physiological body functions and pathological conditions.

The major part of the contributions in this field derives from investigations with four techniques: single-photon emission computerized tomography (SPECT), positron-emission tomography (PET), near-infrared spectroscopy (NIRS) and functional magnetic resonance imaging (fMRI).

All these methods of functional brain imaging rely on the principle that an increase in neuronal activity requires an increase of blood supply [3, 4].

SPECT and PET are two nuclear medicine techniques, which may demonstrate cerebral activity through the accumulation of radioactive substances.

SPECT detects γ-rays emitted by photons. It has a limited temporal and spatial resolution of 10 mm, but it has a lower cost compared to PET.

In PET high-energy photons are produced by the annihilation of the positron-emitting isotopes. The spatial resolution is about 5 mm.

Given that in both nuclear medicine techniques a radioactive substance has to be injected prior to the investigation, they are considered invasive.

NIRS and fMRI rely on the fact that oxygenated and deoxygenated haemoglobin have different physical proprieties. While NIRS signal depends on the fact that oxygenated and deoxygenated haemoglobin have different absorption spectra, fMRI signal basically reflects its different paramagnetic proprieties. Therefore, both techniques are non-invasive.

While NIRS has the lowest spatial resolution (30 mm), its big advantages consist of a high temporal resolution, its low costs and not requiring a strict motion limitation [5, 6].

fMRI has surely established itself as the most feasible, basically given to it being non-invasive and free of radiation. Anyway, even if the last 20 years have seen an explosion of fMRI-based brain imaging studies, this methodology has at least two major limits—to some degree shared with the other techniques.

An intrinsic one lies on the fact that brain structure and circuitry pose a limit on how good fMRI signal can be interpreted. As Logothetis [4] has pointed out, the fMRI signal cannot either be easily differentiated or be easily quantified in its magnitude. In other words, a clear unidirectional discrimination between function-specific processing and neuromodulation, bottom-up and top-down signals, excitation and inhibition as well as brain region activation is not always possible.

A further limit consists of the high variability (if not fragmentation) of the investigation protocols used. Limited consensus exists about the tasks used to investigate brain activity during bladder filling, voiding or urge, while an investigation protocol about voiding in an ecological situation has been defined only few years ago. Procedures may vary according to how fast the bladder is filled, whether and in which position subjects are allowed to void, whether they have to contract or relax the pelvic floor muscle or whether they have to try to suppress urgency, to name a few.

That said, while brain imaging studies represent a very important source of information about brain function the reader should always bear some important caveats in mind:

1. A strong theory about brain function not the data in themselves explains the phenomena observed.
2. Only an integration of data and knowledge coming from different investigative methods (not least anatomical and in vivo studies) can shed light on brain function.

3.3   What Do We Know About the Central Control of Micturition in Healthy Subjects?

3.3.1   Systematizing the Knowledge About Brain and Bladder

In the last decades a growing interest in the investigation of the central control of bladder and micturition has led to many experimental studies as well as many reviews, the latter systematizing the accumulated knowledge in general conceptualizations. In this section the efforts of some authors to derive models of central control of micturition from the data available are presented. The goal of this section is to describe the ongoing evolution of the understanding of central control of micturition.

The neuroimaging studies of today rely on the seminal work of many authors who in the twentieth century investigated the suprapontine control of micturition with methods other than neuroimaging. These authors investigated animal models and pathologies in human patients and were able to formulate important hypotheses which still inform the way we understand the control of micturition.

Examples are represented by the work of Barrington [7], Ueki [8].

What Barrington had described in the cat as "a part of the brain just ventral to the internal edge of the superior cerebellar peduncle from the level of the $V°$ nerve behind to the level of the anterior end of the hind brain in front" has later been referred to as the M-region by Holstege and colleagues [9] and as the pontine micturition centre (PMC) by Loewy and colleagues [10].

Ueki [8] made important observations about micturition in brain tumour patients. In his study he reported that in brain tumours some kind of dysuria (defined as retardation or retardation combined with protraction) was more frequently observed than incontinence. He also stressed the importance of the role played in micturition by the pons, basically confirming Barrington's hypothesis that "there are important centres partaking in contracting the bladder (...) somewhere between the pons and the medulla oblongata, and also close to the lower part of the midbrain".

Until the 1990s there was consensus about the fact that pontine structures were the principal players in micturition control. Later the focus was extended also to suprapontine structures. For example, Blok [11] summarized the components of neural pathways involved in micturition and continence, underlining that "apparently, centers in the pons coordinate micturition as such, but suprapontine centers are responsible for the beginning of micturition". He stressed the important practical observation that "patients with suprapontine lesions never show detrusor-sphincter-dyssynergia".

Later, Fowler and Griffiths presented a "working model of brain activity during bladder filling and emptying" [12].

Basing on the work of Blok [13] these authors underlined the importance of "interoception" defined by Craig [14, 15] as "the sense of the physiological condition of the entire body" which not only is limited to visceral sensation but also comprehends the sensation of pain and temperature. The afferent input regarding these stimuli is conducted through small-diameter ($A\delta$ and C) fibres entering the spinal cord through lamina 1, where lamina 1 neurons relate to homeostatic information. These afferents project to subcortical homeostatic centres (i.e. hypothalamus and PAG) converging—after relaying in the thalamus—on the non-dominant anterior insula. This structure can be seen as the "homeostatic afferent cortex" or "the sensory cortex of the autonomic nervous system" [12] and is activated in a range of tasks involving visceral sensation such as heart rate, respiration, digestive processes and micturition.

Interoceptive sensation is always associated to affective and motivational aspects, which in turn are associated to anterior cingulate cortex (ACC). The ACC can also be seen as "the motor cortex of the autonomic nervous system", given that it is responsible for emotional, behavioural and motor responses to visceral stimuli. Activity in both structures—insula and ACC—has been shown in functional imaging experiments involving the bladder. These structures together with the hypothalamus and the amygdala form the limbic system which is extensively connected with the orbitofrontal or prefrontal lateral cortex, itself involved in "making the decision whether or not micturition should take place".

These data allowed Fowler and Griffiths [12, 16] to describe a "brain bladder control matrix". This matrix involves the following brain structures: brainstem (pons and midbrain), cerebellum, insula and ACC as well as prefrontal cortex (PFC).

Although being a very good attempt to systematize the knowledge about central control of the bladder, this description has two principal limits. On the one hand, it represents a flat map of the structures involved, where connectivity directions are presented as only probable: an attempt to investigate connectivity during visceral interoception has been recently made by Jarrahi and colleagues [17]. On the other hand, it hypothesizes brain activity during bladder filling and emptying, respectively, only generically and in a linear manner.

De Groat and colleagues [18] tried to further differentiate the central control of bladder function, arranging the structures involved in three different circuits.

They are described as follows:

1. The "prefrontal cortex and insula" - involving thalamus, insula, lateral and medial prefrontal cortex and PAG;
2. The "dorsal anterior cingulate cortex and supplemantary motor area" and
3. "Subcortical mechanisms", a network involving PAG and paths of the parahyppocampal cortex.

An attempt to compare the different models drawn from brain imaging data and to show the evolution of the concept is presented in Figs. 3.1 and 3.2.

3.3.2 Structures Involved in the Central Control of the Bladder: The Storage Phase and the Voiding Phase

New methods of neuroimaging meta-analysis such as the activation-likelihood-estimation (ALE) have made it possible the further development of models of central control of the bladder. The ALE method doesn't simply count the brain regions activated during a task but it determines which probability a particular region has to be activated during task execution. It treats each activation focus as a probability distribution which peaks at the reported coordinates. For each voxel the probability

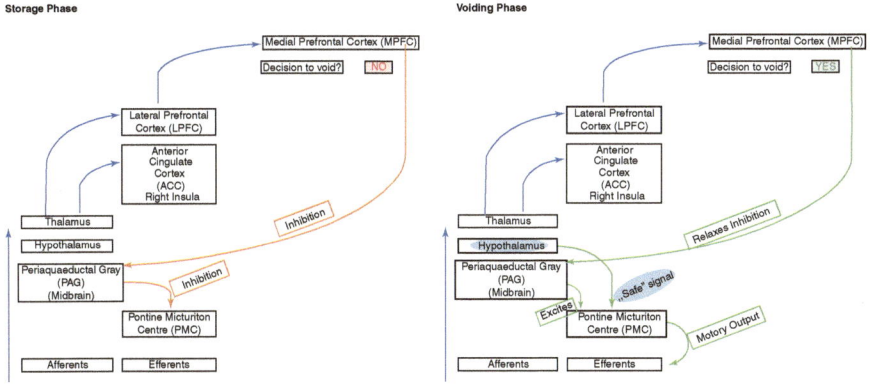

Fig. 3.1 Storage and voiding phases from the model by Fowler and Griffiths [12, 16]

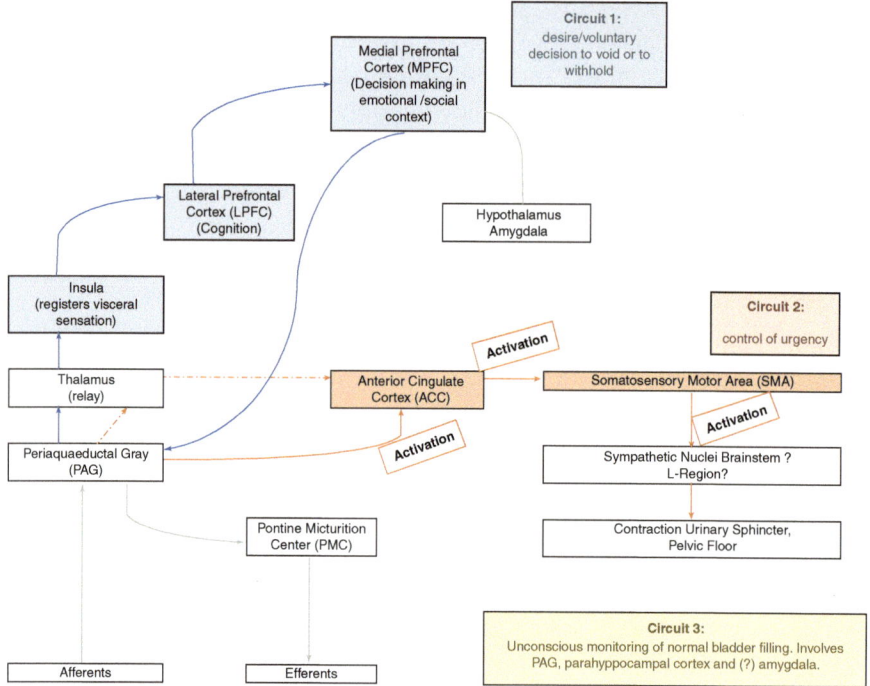

Fig. 3.2 Three circuits involved in bladder control from the model by de Groat, Griffiths and Yoshimura [18]

that at least one of the activation foci lies within it is calculated. The areas of activation are identified, the null hypothesis being the probability that activation foci are spread uniformly throughout the brain.

Two authors have investigated two different phases of bladder control: the storage phase [19] and the voiding phase, respectively [20]. These authors basically confirmed and further systematized the models of bladder control:

3.3.2.1 Brainstem

During the storage phase a cluster activation involving the midbrain and the rostral pons has been identified. In this respect this area in the midbrain probably represented the periaqueductal grey (PAG), which in turn represents the interface between the afferent and the efferent arms of micturition. On the other hand, the activation observed in the pons may reflect the L-region of the pontine micturition centre or the pontine reticular formation, which at least in animal models has been implicated to an inhibitory function on the micturition reflex.

On the other hand, during the voiding phase two different clusters of activation had been observed, with regard to subjects who weren't able to void in the scanner and subjects who were able to do so, the latter showing a more dorsal activation. Nevertheless, it was not possible to ascertain whether those structures represented the pontine micturition and continence centres [19, 20] due to the fact that midbrain images and activity are difficult to acquire via fMRI.

3.3.2.2 Thalamus

The thalamus is a part of the attention and awareness centres, but it also integrates somatosensory information, basically determining which information should reach the cerebral cortex in order to be further processed. Thalamus activation has been observed both during storage and voiding phases. Activation observed during the storage phase may reflect selective attention focused on the signals coming from the bladder. Its activation during the voiding phase may in turn reflect the coordination of the decision to void and the relaxation of the pelvic floor muscle.

3.3.2.3 Cerebellum

Cerebellum activation was observed in both storage and voiding phases. This structure, which plays an important role in motor control, may be involved in the sensory processing of bladder filling—during the storage phase—and in coordinating detrusor contraction with the relaxation of the external urethral sphincter in the voiding phase.

3.3.2.4 Insula and ACC

In the storage phase activation of both insula and ACC was observed. Being a subcortical region where sensory information from the viscera is mapped the insula can be seen as the "seat of interoception" [19]. A right predominating insula activation is observed in healthy controls experiencing normal bladder sensation, with the activation shifting anteriorly during increasing bladder volume and the desire to void becoming stronger.

ACC activation was observed in the storage phase both in healthy controls and in female subjects suffering from overactive bladder (OAB). Given that ACC activation is observed when a strong desire to void is experienced, this can indicate a motor response to the threat of losing urine.

It is less clear why ACC activation in the voiding phase also occurs. Harvie and colleagues [20] suggest two possible explanations: it could point at the importance of afferent signalling to initiate voiding or alternatively it could reflect the tight connection occurring between afferent and efferent centres of the brain.

3.3.2.5 PFC

The PFC is involved in attention networks as well as in the highest brain functions such as executive functions and decision-making. It also has connections to the PAG.

The fact that the bladder is in the storage phase most of the time implies that the PFC has an inhibitory function on the PAG. When a certain threshold is exceeded, afferent signals are sent to the PFC, in order to decide whether voiding is "safe and appropriate" [12]. Only after that the inhibition on the PAG can be lifted and voiding can be initiated. PFC activity was therefore mainly observed during the voiding phase.

3.4 What Do We Know About Pathologies? An Example: Multiple Sclerosis (MS)

In comparison to healthy subjects, MS patients show a lower, more diffused brain activation [21].

An analysis of a large data set of 452 patients showed that the volume of white matter lesions is not solely responsible for disability. The location in itself influences the extent and type of functional disability [22]. On the other hand, functional connectivity in patients unable to void with enhancing lesions was significantly lower in comparison to patients who voided spontaneously [23]. Concerning punctual dysfunctions, MacKenzie-Graham and colleagues [24] observed a significant correlation between loss of grey matter in the right paracentral lobulus and bowel and bladder dysfunction. In MS patients a correlation between neurogenic erectile dysfunction and lesions in the bilateral and predominantly left insula has been observed [25]. Finally, Khavari and colleagues [26] observed that after intradetrusor infiltration of onabotulinumtoxinA in MS-related overactive bladder a modification in the pattern of cerebral activity could be detected.

Now, what are such findings good for? As the authors themselves of the above-mentioned papers stated, the results of their works could have practical implications:

Activation patterns and the quality of BOLD signal activation in certain brain areas may contribute to optimize onabotulinumtoxinA therapy; detection of lesions in the left insular region may help differentiate the origin of erectile dysfunction in male multiple sclerosis patients; the identification of focal lesions or alterations of white mater or connectivity may lead to specific neuroprotective or therapeutic approaches.

Its immediate applicability is still limited, but operators in the field of neurogenic pelvic organ dysfunctions should keep an eye on the evolution of brain imaging.

References

1. Apostolidis A, Wagg A, Rahnam AM, Panicker J, Vrijens D, von Gontard A. Is there "brain OAB" and how can we recognize it? International consultation on incontinence-research society (ICI-RS) 2017. Neurourol Urodyn. 2018;37(S4):S38–45.
2. Sakakibara R, Hattori T, Yasuda K, Yamanishi T. Micturitional disturbance after acute hemispheric stroke: analysis of the lesion site by CT and MRI. J Neurol Sci. 1996;137:47–56.
3. Mosso A. Sulla circolazione del sangue nel cervello dell'uomo. Atti della R Acad Lincei. 1880;III:237–358.
4. Logothetis NK. What we can do and what we cannot do with fMRI. Nature. 2008;435(7197):869–78.

5. Kitta T, Mitsui T, Kanno Z, Chiba H, Moriya K, Shinohara N. Brain-bladder control network: The unsolved 21st century urological mystery. Int J Urol. 2015;22(4):342–8.
6. Committee on the mathematics and physics of emerging dynamic biomedical imaging, mathematics and physics of emerging biomedical imaging, National Academies Press; 1996. http://www.nap.edu/catalog/5066.html. Accessed 20 Jun 2019.
7. Barrington F. The effect of lesions of the hind- and mid-brain on micturition in the cat. Q J Exp Physiol. 1925;15:81–102.
8. Ueki K. Disturbances of micturition observed in some patients with brain tumour. Neurol Med Chir. 1960;2:25–33.
9. Holstege G, Kuypers H, Boer R. Anatomical evidence for direct brainstem projections to the somatic motoneuronal cell groups and autonomic preganglionic cell groups in cat spinal cord. Brain Res. 1979;171(2):329–33.
10. Loewy A, Saper C, Baker R. Descending projections from the pontine micturition center. Brain Res. 1979;172(3):533–8.
11. Blok BF. Central Pathways controlling micturition and urinary continence. Urology. 2002;59(5 Suppl 1):13–7.
12. Fowler CJ, Griffiths DJ. A decade of functional brain imaging applied to bladder control. Neurourol Urodyn. 2010;29(1):49–55.
13. Blok BF, Willemsen AT, Holstege G. A PET study on brain control of micturition in humans. Brain. 1997;120(Pt 1):11–121.
14. Craig AD. How do you feel? Interoception: the sense of physiologic al condition of the body. Nat Rev Neurosci. 2002;3(8):655–66.
15. Craig AD. Interoception: the sense of the physiological condition of the body. Curr Opin Neurobiol. 2003;13(4):500–5.
16. Fowler CJ, Griffiths D, de Groat WC. The neural control of micturition. Nat Rev Neurosci. 2008;9(6):453–66.
17. Jarrahi B, Mantini D, Balsters JH, Michels L, Kessler TM, Mehnert U, et al. Differential functional brain network connectivity during visceral interoception as revealed by independent component analysis of fMRI TIME-series. Hum Brain Mapp. 2015;36(11):4438–68.
18. de Groat W, Griffiths D, Yoshimura N. Neural control of the lower urinary tract. Compr Physiol. 2015;5(1):327–96.
19. Arya N, Weissbart S, Xu S, Rao H. Brain activation in response to bladder filling in healthy adults: an activation likelihood estimation meta-analysis of neuroimaging studies. Neurourol Urodyn. 2017;36(4):960–5.
20. Harvie C, Weissbart SJ, Priyanka KA, Rao H, Arya LA. Brain activation during the voiding phase of micturition in healthy adults: a meta-analysis of neuroimaging studies. Clin Anat. 2019;32(1):13–9.
21. Khavari R, Karmonik C, Shy M, Fletcher S, Boone T. Functional magnetic resonance imaging with concurrent urodynamic testing identifies brain structures involved in micturition cycle in patients with multiple sclerosis. J Urol. 2017;197(2):438–44.
22. Charil A, Zijdenbos A, Taylor J, Boelman C, Worsley K, Evans A, et al. Statistical mapping analysis of lesion location and neurological disability in multiple sclerosis: application to 452 patient data sets. NeuroImage. 2003;19(3):532–4.
23. Khavari R, Elias S, Boone T, Karmonik C. Similarity of functional connectivity patterns in patients with multiple sclerosis who void spontaneously versus patients with voiding dysfunction. Neurourol Urodyn. 2019;38(1):239–47.
24. MacKenzie-Graham A, Kurth F, Itoh Y, Wang H, Montag M, Elashoff R, et al. Disability-specific atlases of gray matter loss in relapsing-remitting multiple sclerosis. JAMA Neurol. 2016;73(8):944–53.
25. Winder K, Linker R, Seifert F, Deutsch M, Engelhorn T, Dörfler A, et al. Insular multiple sclerosis lesions are associated with erectile dysfunction. J Neurol. 2018;265(4):783–92.
26. Khavari R, Elias S, Pande R, Wu K, Boone T, Karmonik C. Higher neural correlates in patients with multiple sclerosis and neurogenic overactive bladder following treatment with intradetrusor injection of onabotulinumtoxin. J Urol. 2019;201(1):135–40.

Urodynamic Patterns and Prevalence of N-LUTDs in Suprapontine Lesions

4

Eugenia Fragalà

4.1 Introduction

The prevalence of NLUTD in SPL is quite uncertain due to the poor number of epidemiology studies and the heterogeneity of the populations studied. Again, few data are reported in literature stratifying and analyzing patients with SPL.

Several SPL can affect the lower urinary tract function and lead to several lower urinary tract symptoms (LUTS) which may onset acutely or gradually according to the type of injury whether traumatic or not, stable or progressive (Fig. 4.1).

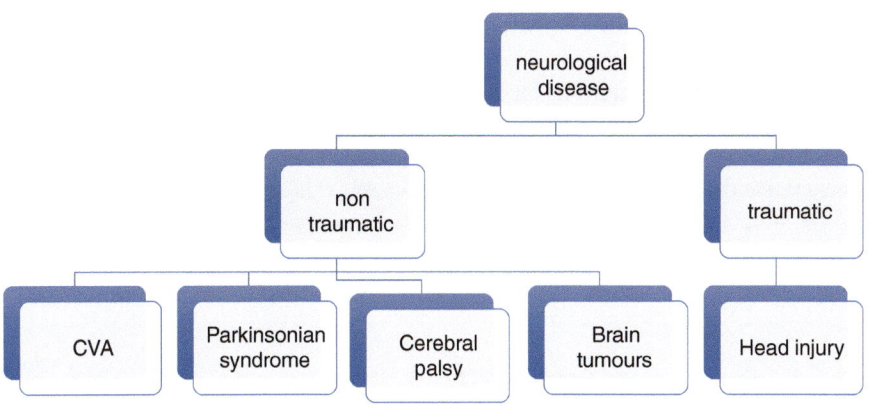

Fig. 4.1 Neurological disease classification

E. Fragalà (✉)

Department of Urology, Hospital G.B. Morgagni- L. Pierantoni of Forlí, Forlí-Cesena, Italy

e-mail: dr.eugenia.fragala@outlook.com

© Springer Nature Switzerland AG 2020

G. Lamberti et al. (eds.), *Suprapontine Lesions and Neurogenic Pelvic Dysfunctions*, Urodynamics, Neurourology and Pelvic Floor Dysfunctions, https://doi.org/10.1007/978-3-030-29775-6_4

4.2   Cerebrovascular Accident (Stroke)

Stroke incidence ranges from 41 to 316 per 100,000 persons per year [1]; between stroke survivors only 10% have no residual effects, whereas 40% have mild disability, 40% have significant disability, and 10% require nursing home care [2].

NLUTDs are considered as one of the most affecting factors on health-related quality of life in poststroke patients [3]. Prevalence of urological complaints after cerebrovascular accidents (CVAs) ranges from 11% to almost 80% [4].

Urinary incontinence is the most common sequela of stroke [2, 5]. Patients may also report nocturia (36–79%), frequency (17.5–36%), urgency (19–29%), difficulty in voiding (25%), straining (3.5%), and pain (2.5%) [6–8]. Of course, the symptom presentation depends on the stroke phase.

In the acute phase of CVAs patients often show urinary retention that can be a neural representation of brain infract ("cerebral shock") and manifests as neurogenic detrusor underactivity (NDU) or a nonrelaxing/overactive pelvic floor function.

In the post-acute (chronic) phase of stroke, normal bladder function can return or impaired bladder function may evolve to a chronic and usually stable dysfunction, mainly manifested by frequency and urgency and urgency incontinence [2].

The presence of NLUTDs following stroke has been strongly associated with increased mortality rates, poor functional outcomes, and worse health-related quality of life [9].

4.3   Parkinsonian Syndrome

The "Parkinsonian syndrome" includes a number of various nosologic entities that are grouped together on the basis of their shared clinical features but are separated on the basis of their different pathologies [10]. It is the second prevalent neurodegenerative disease after the Alzheimer's disease [11].

A simple classification system splits Parkinsonian syndrome into Parkinson's disease (75–80%) and non-Parkinson's disease (20% with the greatest prevalence of multiple system atrophy).

4.3.1   Parkinson's Disease (PD)

About 70% of PD patients suffer from NLUTDs [12] which commonly worse with the progression of the neurological disease. A multinational survey of 545 patients with a mild PD showed that patients usually report nocturia (62%) and urgency with or without incontinence (56%) [13]; less common are instead the voiding symptoms such as hesitancy, straining to void, and poor urinary stream, especially in the initial stages of the disease. Post-void residuals are typically low [14]; nevertheless it is necessary to remember the possible coexistence of bladder outlet obstruction (BOO) due for instance to benign prostatic hyperplasia (BPH) in elderly PD patients.

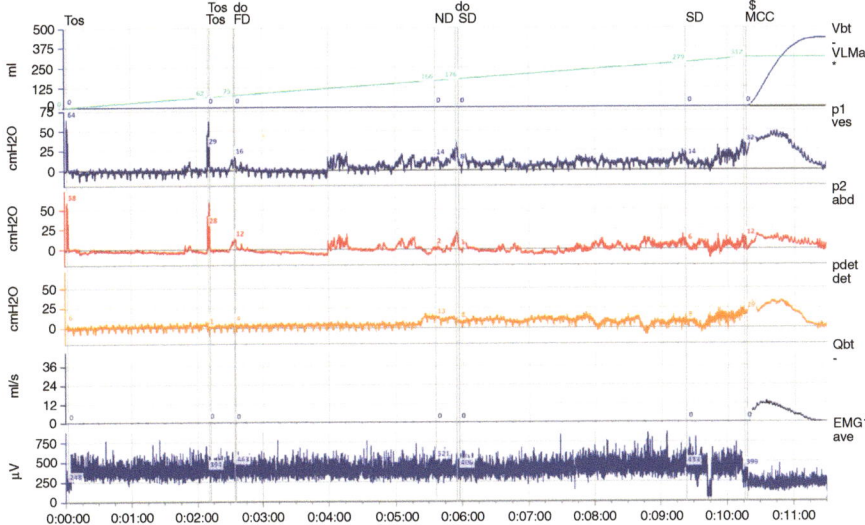

Fig. 4.2 Male 70 years old affected by PD. UD: detrusor overactivity, preserved bladder sensation

NDO with preserved bladder sensation is the most common urodynamic finding in patients with PD which are described in 36–93% of all cases (Fig. 4.2) [12]. NDU or acontractile detrusor may also be found (0–48%). Some studies demonstrated the evolution of the bladder behavior from NDO to NDU accordingly to the disease progression [15]. Majority of studies have reported a sphincter bradykinesia suggesting that an impaired or a delayed relaxation of the striated sphincter might exist although it is not defined as a proper dyssynergia [14, 16, 17].

4.3.2 Multiple System Atrophy (MSA)

Almost all of the patients (up to 96%) having MSA report urinary symptoms [18]. The commonest urinary symptom which is also considered a clinical parameter differentiating MSA from PD patients is voiding difficulty (79%), followed by storage symptoms such as nocturia (74%), urgency (63%), incontinence (63%), frequency (45%), nocturnal enuresis (19%), and urinary retention (8%). Patients may also show a combination of these symptoms. Up to 50–60% of MSA patients develop LUTS either before or concomitantly with orthostatic symptoms or motor disorders [19].

Considering urodynamics, NDO can be observed in 33–100% of patients with MSA, whereas NDU may be reported in 60% (Fig. 4.3) [19]. A subgroup of patients with MSA may show NDO during storage and NDU during voiding phase. Since MSA affects multiple brain regions, even the pons and lower regions, also a true detrusor-sphincter dyssynergia (DSD) is described in 47% of MSA patients [20, 21]; moreover 46–100% of MSA patients may show open bladder neck reflecting

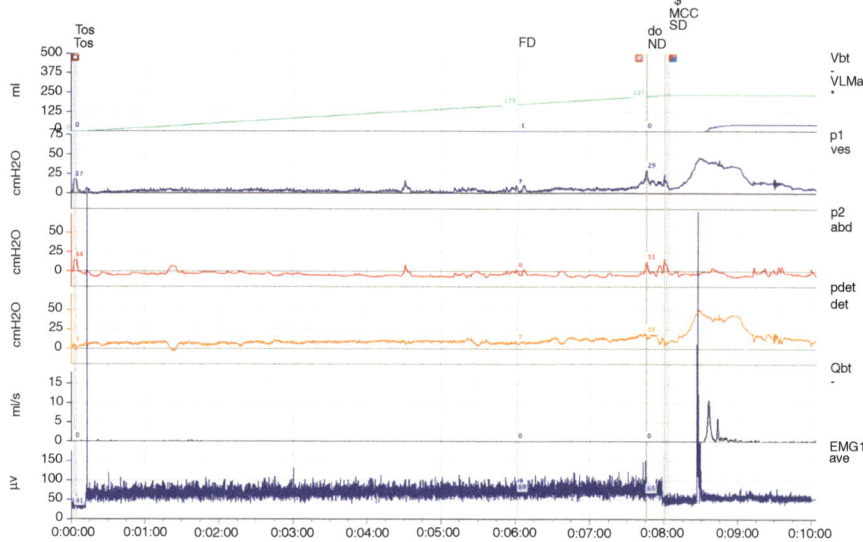

Fig. 4.3 Female 64 years old affected by MSA. UD: detrusor overactivity and detrusor hypocontractility

the intrinsic sphincter deficiency with urinary incontinence [20]. Uninhibited relaxation of the external sphincter may also be occasionally found during the filling phase and results in exacerbation of urinary incontinence.

4.4   Dementia

Dementia is a general term to describe a decline in mental ability which interferes with daily life; it affects 6.4% of adults over 65 years [22].

Alzheimer's disease (AD) is the most prevalent irreversible cause of dementia (around 60–80% of cases).

LUTS may occur especially in the later phases of illness. Urinary incontinence is the most frequent symptom with a prevalence rate of 11–90% [23], although its etiology seems to be not only secondary to the underlying neurological illness, but also multifactorial including cognitive and physical disabilities, impaired conscious willingness, comorbidities, and surrounding environment.

4.5   Brain Tumors

Intracranial tumor incidence rate is about 10.82 per 100,000 individuals [24].

Brain tumors impair central voiding regulation. Urinary incontinence is the most frequent symptom and occurs in frontal located brain tumors and it is part of the frontal syndrome. Tumors in the frontal lobe may cause a loss of the central inhibitory output and lead to detrusor overactivity with urge incontinence. Voluntary control of voiding may also be impaired.

The incidence of LUTS among patients with frontal lobe tumors has been estimated as 14–28% [25].

Patients typically report storage symptoms like urgency, frequency, nocturia, and incontinence but symptom presentation can vary. Patients with pontine tumors are more likely to have voiding difficulties and retention.

Data on urodynamic findings in patients with intracranial tumors are scant and limited to single studies or case reports.

4.6   Cerebral Palsy

Cerebral palsy ranges from 3.1 to 3.6/1000 in children aged 8 years [26].

Approximately of 55.5% of subjects with CP experience one or more LUTS [27]. Urinary incontinence is the most frequent symptom with a prevalence ranging between 20 and 94%. Urgency and frequency are also reported in 38.5% and 22.5% of patients, respectively. Voiding symptoms are less prevalent than storage problems. Prevalence rate of hesitancy varies between 2 and 51.5%, with an average of 24%.

NDO is the commonest urodynamic observation, with a mean prevalence rate of 59% although more than 44% of CP patients having NDO do not report LUTS [28, 29]. About 70% of subjects with CP also show a reduced bladder capacity compared to the expected bladder capacity for age. Interestingly, some studies report DSD in 11% [27]. As CP definition includes only suprapontine insult, this peculiar finding may be explained in some patients as a concomitant unrevealed spinal lesion. Another theory stresses that investigated DSD is indeed a pseudo-DSD resulting from pelvic floor overactivity as a voluntary reaction to bladder overactivity.

4.7   Head Injury

Traumatic brain injuries affect suprapontine structures, often leading to NDO. Studies suggest that NDO is prevalently associated with right-side damage [30, 31], whereas left hemispheric injury is linked to impaired contractility [32]. Frontal lobe injuries determine NLUTDs more than injuries of other lobes [33, 34]; unilateral right cortical lesions in the prefrontal area produce temporary dysfunction; instead bilateral lesions are inclined to provoke permanent and chronic NLUTDs [35].

In the acute phase of traumatic brain injury spontaneous micturition is possible with persistent perception of bladder fullness; in mild stages [36, 37], voiding function is synergistic, with no pathological post-void residual (PVR). However, in up to 10% of acute patients, retention may be observed and the exact mechanism of this dysfunction has not been well investigated [38].

In post-acute phase, patients mainly report frequency, urgency, and urgency incontinence.

Symptom severity is usually in line with the extent of the injury [33]. PVR is not pathologic as a result of involuntary detrusor contractions [31].

Finally, NDO and a normal external sphincter function are the urodynamic patterns most frequently observed [39], although in some cases a reduced detrusor compliance has been described [33].

4.8 Conclusion

The wideness of the different SPL compromising distinct anatomic structure involved in the micturition control, the different types of neurological evolution during time (acute, chronic, progressive SPL), the possible presence of concomitant comorbidities due to the age of this population, or the presence of secondary neurological factors such as cognitive impairments are still the greatest challenges of knowledge which may amplify the clinical and urodynamic pitfalls in the diagnosis of NLUTDs in these subjects. Future research in neuro-urology should dedicate more interest to reduce this gap and help all clinicians to ameliorate continence care in SPL patients.

References

1. Feigin VL, Krishnamurthi RV, Parmar P, Norrving B, Mensah GA, Bennett DA, et al. Update on the global burden of ischemic and hemorrhagic stroke in 1990–2013: the GBD 2013 study. Neuroepidemiology. 2015;45(3):161–76.
2. Osborn DJ, Reynolds WS, Dmochowski RR. Cerebrovascular accidents, intracranial tumors, and urologic consequences. In: Corcos J, Ginsberg D, Karsenty G, editors. Textbook of the neurogenic bladder. 3rd ed. Boca Raton: CRC Press/Taylor & Francis; 2016. p. 260–4.
3. Tapia CI, Khalaf K, Berenson K, Globe D, Chancellor M, Carr LK. Health-related quality of life and economic impact of urinary incontinence due to detrusor overactivity associated with a neurologic condition: a systematic review. Health Qual Life Outcomes. 2013;11:13.
4. Ruffion A, Castro-Diaz D, Patel H, Khalaf K, Onyenwenyi A, Globe D, et al. Systematic review of the epidemiology of urinary incontinence and detrusor overactivity among patients with neurogenic overactive bladder. Neuroepidemiology. 2013;41(3–4):146–55.
5. Mehdi Z, Birns J, Bhalla A. Post-stroke urinary incontinence. Int J Clin Pract. 2013;67(11):1128–37.
6. Brittain KR, Perry SI, Peet SM, Shaw C, Dallosso H, Assassa RP, et al. Prevalence and impact of urinary symptoms among community-dwelling stroke survivors. Stroke. 2000;31(4): 886–91.
7. Sakakibara R, Hattori T, Yasuda K, Yamanishi T. Micturitional disturbance after acute hemispheric stroke: analysis of the lesion site by CT and MRI. J Neurol Sci. 1996;137(1):47–56.
8. Williams MP, Srikanth V, Bird M, Thrift AG. Urinary symptoms and natural history of urinary continence after first-ever stroke—a longitudinal population-based study. Age Ageing. 2012;41(3):371–6.
9. Rotar M, Blagus R, Jeromel M, Skrbec M, Trsinar B, Vodusek DB. Stroke patients who regain urinary continence in the first week after acute first-ever stroke have better prognosis than patients with persistent lower urinary tract dysfunction. Neurourol Urodyn. 2011;30(7):1315–8.
10. Williams DR, Litvan I. Parkinsonian syndromes. Continuum (Minneap Minn). 2013;19(5 Movement Disorders):1189–212.

11. Pringsheim T, et al. The prevalence of Parkinson's disease: a systematic review and meta-analysis. Mov Disord. 2014;29:15883.
12. Ogawa T, Seki S, Yoshimura N, et al. Pathologies of basal ganglia, such as Parkinson's and Huntington's diseases. In: Corcos J, Ginsberg D, Karsenty G, editors. Textbook of the neurogenic bladder. 3rd ed. Boca Raton: CRC Press/Taylor & Francis; 2016. p. 199–207.
13. Martinez-Martin P, Schapira AH, Stocchi F, Sethi K, Odin P, MacPhee G, et al. Prevalence of nonmotor symptoms in Parkinson's disease in an international setting; study using nonmotor symptoms questionnaire in 545 patients. Mov Disord. 2007;22(11):1623–9.
14. Sakakibara R, Kishi M, Ogawa E, Tateno F, Uchiyama T, Yamamoto T, Yamanishi T. Bladder, bowel, and sexual dysfunction in Parkinson's disease. Parkinsons Dis. 2011;2011:924605. https://doi.org/10.4061/2011/924605.
15. Araki I, Kuno S. Assessment of voiding dysfunction in Parkinson's disease by the international prostate symptom score. J Neurol Neurosurg Psychiatry. 2000;68(4):429–33.
16. Pavlakis AJ, Siroky MB, Goldstein I, Krane RJ. Neurourologic findings in Parkinson's disease. J Urol. 1983;129(1):80–3.
17. Stocchi F, Carbone A, Inghilleri M, Monge A, Ruggieri S, Berardelli A, et al. Urodynamic and neurophysiological evaluation in Parkinson's disease and multiple system atrophy. J Neurol Neurosurg Psychiatry. 1997;62(5):507–11.
18. Sakakibara R, Hattori T, Uchiyama T, Kita K, Asahina M, Suzuki A, et al. Urinary dysfunction and orthostatic hypotension in multiple system atrophy: which is the more common and earlier manifestation? J Neurol Neurosurg Psychiatry. 2000;68(1):65–9.
19. Ogawa T, Sakakibara R, Kuno S, Ishizuka O, Kitta T, Yoshimura N. Prevalence and treatment of LUTS in patients with Parkinson disease or multiple system atrophy. Nat Rev Urol. 2017;14(2):79–89.
20. Sakakibara R, Hattori T, Uchiyama T, Yamanishi T. Videourodynamic and sphincter motor unit potential analyses in Parkinson's disease and multiple system atrophy. J Neurol Neurosurg Psychiatry. 2001;71(5):600–6.
21. Blaivas JG, Sinha HP, Zayed AA, Labib KB. Detrusor-external sphincter dyssynergia: a detailed electromyographic study. J Urol. 1981;125(4):545–8.
22. Lobo A, et al. Prevalence of dementia and major subtypes in Europe: a collaborative study of population-based cohorts. Neurologic diseases in the elderly research group. Neurology. 2000;54:S4.
23. Sakakibara R. Dementia and lower urinary tract dysfunction. In: Corcos J, Ginsberg D, Karsenty G, editors. Textbook of the neurogenic bladder. 3rd ed. Boca Raton: CRC Press/Taylor & Francis; 2016. p. 179–99.
24. De Robles P, Fiest KM, Frolkis AD, Pringsheim T, Atta C, St Germaine-Smith C, et al. The worldwide incidence and prevalence of primary brain tumors: a systematic review and meta-analysis. Neuro-Oncology. 2015;17(6):776–83.
25. Sakakibara R. Lower urinary tract dysfunction in patients with brain lesions. Handb Clin Neurol. 2015;130:269–87.
26. Dolecek TA, et al. CBTRUS statistical report: primary brain and central nervous system tumors diagnosed in the United States in 2005-2009. Neuro Oncol. 2012;14(Suppl 5):v1–49.
27. Samijn B, Van Laecke E, Renson C, Hoebeke P, Plasschaert F, Vande Walle J, et al. Lower urinary tract symptoms and urodynamic findings in children and adults with cerebral palsy: a systematic review. Neurourol Urodyn. 2017;36(3):541–9.
28. Chiu PK, Yam KY, Lam TY, Cheng CH, Yu C, Li ML, et al. Does selective dorsal rhizotomy improve bladder function in children with cerebral palsy? Int Urol Nephrol. 2014;46(10):1929–33.
29. Delialioglu SU, Culha C, Tunc H, et al. Evaluation of lower urinary system symptoms and neurogenic bladder in children with cerebral palsy: relationships with the severity of cerebral palsy and mental status. Turk J Med Sci. 2009;39:571–8.
30. Kuroiwa Y, Tohgi H, Ono S, Itoh M. Frequency and urgency of micturition in hemiplegic patients: relationship to hemisphere laterality of lesions. J Neurol. 1987;234(2):100–2.

31. Singhania P, Andankar MG, Pathak HR. Urodynamic evaluation of urinary disturbances following traumatic brain injury. Urol Int. 2010;84(1):89–93.
32. Giannantoni A, Silvestro D, Siracusano S, Azicnuda E, D'Ippolito M, Rigon J, et al. Urologic dysfunction and neurologic outcome in coma survivors after severe traumatic brain injury in the post-acute and chronic phase. Arch Phys Med Rehabil. 2011;92(7):1134–8.
33. Moiyadi AV, Devi BI, Nair KP. Urinary disturbances following traumatic brain injury: clinical and urodynamic evaluation. NeuroRehabilitation. 2007;22(2):93–8.
34. Oostra K, Everaert K, Van Laere M. Urinary incontinence in brain injury. Brain Inj. 1996;10(6):459–64.
35. Mochizuki H, Saito H. Mesial frontal lobe syndrome: correlations between neurological deficits and radiological localizations. Tohoku J Exp Med. 1990;161(Suppl):231–9.
36. Wyndaele J. Urodynamics in comatose patients. Neurourol Urodyn. 1990;9:43–52.
37. Wyndaele JJ. Micturition in comatose patients. J Urol. 1986;135(6):1209–11.
38. Chua K, Chuo A, Kong KH. Urinary incontinence after traumatic brain injury: incidence, outcomes and correlates. Brain Inj. 2003;17(6):469–78.
39. Krimchansky BZ, Sazbon L, Heller L, Kosteff H, Luttwak Z. Bladder tone in patients in post-traumatic vegetative state. Brain Inj. 1999;13(11):899–903.

Suprapontine Lesions and Neurogenic Pelvic Dysfunctions

5

Julien Renard, Eugenia Fragalà, Gianfranco Lamberti,
Federica Petraglia, Francesco Verderosa, Anna Cassio,
and Giovanni Panariello

5.1 Cerebrovascular Accidents (CVAs)

When considering cerebrovascular accident lower urinary tract symptoms (LUTS) are very frequent in the acute phase. The main symptoms consist of storage symptoms: incontinence has been reported in 32–79% of stroke patients admitted to hospitals with up to 25% of them remaining incontinent at 1 year. Patients may also report nocturia (36–79%), frequency (17.5–36%), urgency (19–29%), difficulty in

J. Renard (✉)
Divison of Urology, Geneva University Hospital, Geneva, Switzerland

Division of Neuro-Urology, Ente Ospedaliera Cantonale -Ospedale Regionale di Bellinzona and Ospedale Italiano di Lugano, Lugano, Switzerland

E. Fragalà
Department of Urology, Hospital G.B. Morgagni- L. Pierantoni of Forlí, Forlí-Cesena, Italy
e-mail: dr.eugenia.fragala@outlook.com

G. Lamberti
Neurorehabilitation Unit and Pelvic Floor Dysfunction Rehabilitation Center,
SS Trinità Hospital, Cuneo, Italy

F. Petraglia
Physical Medicine and Rehabilitation Residency Program, University of Parma, Parma, Italy

F. Verderosa
Spinal Unit and Intensive Rehabilitation Medicine A.U.S.L. Piacenza,
Emilia Romagna Region, Italy
e-mail: f.verderosa@ausl.pc.it

A. Cassio
Spinal Unit AUSL Piacenza, Piacenza, Italy
e-mail: A.CASSIO@ausl.pc.it

G. Panariello
Unit of Physical and Rehabilitation Medicine, Local Health Authority (ASL) of Avellino,
Avellino, Italy

© Springer Nature Switzerland AG 2020
G. Lamberti et al. (eds.), *Suprapontine Lesions and Neurogenic Pelvic Dysfunctions*, Urodynamics, Neurourology and Pelvic Floor Dysfunctions,
https://doi.org/10.1007/978-3-030-29775-6_5

voiding (25%), straining (3.5%), and pain (2.5%) [2, 3]. It is important however to point out that there is a great difficulty to assess correctly LUTS directly caused by the neurological insult. In fact, patients who suffer from stroke usually tend to already present LUT disorder acting as a confounder. In a nationwide population study recently published this matter was addressed. It demonstrated that male stroke patients experienced more LUTS including both voiding (straining, weak stream, intermittency and incomplete emptying) and storage symptoms (frequency, urgency and nocturia) than male non-stroke patients. Importantly stroke was found to be an independent risk factor even after adjusting for the confounding factors that potentially affect LUTS.

It is also important to point out that symptoms will decrease in the months following the acute neurological event (6–12 months). Some data would suggest a higher frequency of UI in the presence of anterior cerebral ischemic or haemorrhagic lesions rather than of occipital lesions. The prognostic interpretation of incontinence remains controversial too: according to some authors, its appearance within 1 week from the onset of the stroke is an unfavourable element for recovery and a predictor of an inauspicious outcome at 6 and 12 months from the acute event [4]. This data may be conditioned by not considering the presence of UI prior to the stroke, thus having an epidemiologically incorrect observation. In a specular manner, the improvement of urinary incontinence or its absence is associated with a more favourable outcome and in any case, in 50% of cases, the reduction in episodes of UI is correlated with clinical improvement in general (autonomy, mobility, cognitive component) [5]. This implies the need for initial conservative treatment. In the case of patients requiring surgery after stroke for bladder outlet obstruction (mostly BPH) preoperative urodynamic examination is mandatory as bladder diaries or non-invasive diagnostic tools might not detect all abnormalities present. If patient undergoes surgery, he should be warned that functional results are frequently bad and may potentially worsen the actual situation [6–9].

Constipation and faecal incontinence are frequent in the outcomes of cerebrovascular disease and weigh heavily on the quality of life of these persons. Constipation appears to be constantly present both in the acute phase, regardless of the physical activity allowed and the side of the lesion, and months after the acute event [10].

People with haemorrhagic lesions would appear to be more susceptible to constipation than those affected by ischemic stroke.

Less significant are the data in the literature on incidence and risk factors for faecal incontinence after acquired brain injury: during the acute phase the incidence varies between 23% and 68% with a hypothesised persistence in the chronic phase between 5% and 15% of patients; more generally, during a chronic phase, more than 20% of people with brain lesions complain of constipation [11].

Diarrhoea also, a frequent cause of faecal incontinence, is a common complication of dysbiosis secondary to enteral nutrition and to the other treatments which are often necessary during the acute phase (e.g. antibiotics, beta blockers). The late onset of FI in case of a stroke (often caused by overflow) may be affected by the loss of motor autonomy in going to the toilet and is frequently associated with UI, which is a strong predictor [12].

Regarding sexual activity, the incidence of erectile dysfunction (ED) post-stroke ranges from 26% to 60%. Changes in libido occurred in 44–70% of overall patients with significant reduction of vaginal lubrication in females. Sexual dissatisfaction and dysfunction were seen also at 2-year follow-up after the acute event. Of course comorbidities such as psychological aspects can affect sexual function as well as loss of libido was found to be predictive of depression. No conclusive data are reported regarding the possible correlation with the hemispheric lesioned side [13].

5.2 Traumatic Brain Injury

LUTS can also be observed in the aftermath of traumatic brain injury. Symptoms are usually caused by midbrain dysfunction secondary to compression, ischaemia or haemorrhage and the primary traumatic lesion. It has also been described that there is a direct relationship between urinary incontinence and severity of neurologic outcome [14, 15].

Urinary retention is often correlated with severe constipation; prolonged bed confinement promotes loss of functionality of the abdominal muscles, accentuating the slower transit. It seems that the presence of faeces in the rectal ampulla can influence the morphology of the bladder-urethral angle, facilitating mechanical urinary retention [16].

Modifications in sexual activity including ED and loss of libido but also paraphilic and hypersexual disorders are described in more than one-third of patients with a consequent negative impact on their couples' relationship and partner/spouse sexual functioning [17, 18].

5.3 Normal-Pressure Hydrocephalus

Normal-pressure hydrocephalus is a condition affecting older adults. Incidence has reached in various studies up to 20 million people [19]. This condition is characterized by a triad (Hakim's triad) composed of dementia, gait disturbance and urinary incontinence. Most of these patients will present overactive bladder symptoms in 64% of cases with urodynamic evidence of detrusor activity in 95% of cases often associated to incontinence (~54% of cases) and to bladder outlet obstruction. The underlying pathophysiology seems to be decreased cerebral blood flow in the right frontal cortex, and to a lesser extent altered basal ganglia function. Urinary incontinence can overlap the detrusor overactivity to impaired cognition/initiative, immobility or disturbed consciousness in this disorder [20].

Treatment of cause through cerebro-fluid shunt could resolve LUTS [21]. Conversely, enterocutaneous fistulae, bowel obstruction and/or perforation could occur as acute or later complications of ventriculus-peritoneal catheter positioning [22].

5.4   Cerebral Palsy

Cerebral palsy is a disorder of the development of movement and posture, causing activity limitations attributed to non-progressive disturbances of the foetal or infant brain that may also affect sensation, perception, cognition, communication and behaviour.

Motor control during reaching, grasping and walking is disturbed by spasticity, dyskinesia, hyperreflexia, excessive coactivation of antagonist muscles, retained developmental reactions and secondary musculoskeletal malformations, together with paresis and defective programming [23]. Its prevalence is roughly 3.1–3.6 in every 1000 children with aetiologies including prematurity, foetal hypoxia and maternal infection during gestation. The cerebral insult removes inhibitory control over the pontine micturition centre and results in a high prevalence of neurogenic detrusor overactivity [24].

Urinary incontinence is the most frequently observed LUTS with a prevalence ranging between 20% and 94%. This condition is usually linked to neurogenic detrusor activity, but other risk factors are functional impairment, intellectual disability and oral fluid intake. Treatment should therefore include in adjunction to medical treatment and management of bladder dysfunction strategies to minimize the impact of these additional risk factors in order to achieve continence [25].

The mean daytime bladder and bowel continence in bilateral CP children has been observed to be slower compared to healthy children (5.4 vs. 2.4 years). Only about half of bilateral CP subjects achieve night-time bladder and bowel continence when 12–14 years old [26].

Also, dating and intimate relationships are significantly delayed in CP adolescents although secondary sexual characteristics and puberty maturation usually start and end earlier than their age-race-matched mates [27].

5.5   Brain Tumour (BT)

Intracranial mass lesions can also be the cause of lower urinary tract symptom. The literature accounts for different reports of urinary frequency, urgency and urinary incontinence in association with frontal lobe lesion with some cases having the onset of LUTS as the first symptom of a brain mass [28].

No data are reported in literature regarding the bowel function in BT. One possible reason could be the high rate of bowel adverse events secondary to the oncological treatment such as chemo- and/or radiotherapy which makes the evaluation during follow-up difficult.

5.6   Parkinsonian Syndrome

5.6.1 Parkinson's Disease

Most of Parkinson's disease (PD) patients (up to 70%) suffer from bladder dysfunctions. Bladder symptoms worsen as the disease advances. A multinational survey of 545 patients with mild PD showed that patients usually report nocturia (62%) and urgency with or without incontinence (56%); less common are the voiding symptoms, represented by hesitancy, straining to void and poor urinary stream, particularly in advanced stages of the disease. LUTS may be induced by the reduction of the inhibitory effects of dopamine D1 receptors although it is worth mentioning the possible coexistence of benign prostatic hyperplasia as a confounder factor for the diagnosis and the following achievement of treatment success in PD elderly patients [29–32].

When affected by PD, the whole gastrointestinal tract is compromised, with a general prevalence of approximately 50% and of constipation (between 30% and 80%), diarrhoea (~25%) and faecal incontinence (10–20%). Constipation may be related to the degeneration of the dopaminergic pathways, but also to a more general impairment of the parasympathetic system [33].

The reduced passage of the faecal bolus in the rectum and the abdominal-pelvic dyssynergia can be interpreted in this sense; faecal incontinence in some cases is caused by overflow, caused by the difficulty in emptying the anorectum [34, 35].

A progressive reduction of sexual activity from 56.3% to 50.8% has been described in men, mainly ED, and over the 2-year follow-up since the early stage of PD and this seems to be correlated with reduced motor and non-motor burden. Women are almost twice sexually inactive than men (33% vs. 67%). Female sexual dysfunction seems to mostly depend on urinary incontinence [36].

5.6.2 Multiple System Atrophy

Almost overall (up to 96%) multiple system atrophy (MSA) patients report urinary symptoms. The most frequently reported urinary symptom is voiding difficulty (79%), followed by nocturia (74%), urgency (63%), incontinence (63%), frequency (45%), nocturnal enuresis (19%) and urinary retention (8%). Patients may also present with a combination of these symptoms. Up to 50–60% of patients with MSA develop urinary symptoms either before or around the time of presentation with orthostatic symptoms or motor disorders [31, 32].

Compared with the PD the prevalence and severity of urinary and bowel dysfunction are significantly higher for urinary urgency (76% in MSA vs. 58 in PD), hesitation (79% vs. 48%) and constipation (58% vs. 31%) [37].

5.7 Unresponsive Wakefulness Syndrome

Following a severe vascular or traumatic cerebrovascular lesion, a disturbance of the state of consciousness may arise, initially classifiable as a coma; the latter is fundamentally characterised by the absence of spontaneous eye opening and by the absence of reaction to any stimulus, even painful (absence of wakefulness), and by the absence of self-awareness and of the surrounding environment.

The state of coma is usually transient and evolves into the state of unresponsive wakefulness, where the affected person appears spontaneously open-eyed although without any consciousness of himself/herself and of the surrounding environment.

A further evolution can be detected in the state of minimal consciousness, at the moment in which contact with the environment, appropriate emotional responses to external stimuli and functional use of objects appear consistently.

Urinary and intestinal dysfunctions have not been particularly studied in the case of disorders of the state of consciousness either. Urodynamic studies performed on small samples almost always showed a picture of detrusor hyperactivity with bladder detrusor-sphincter synergy [38, 39].

This data has also been highlighted in animal models where bladder dysfunction changes from underactive to overactive after experimental traumatic brain injury in rats.

In the absence of a concomitant cord lesion, the urinary reflex is therefore basically maintained in these patients [40, 41].

References

1. Holstege G. Micturition and the soul. J Comp Neurol. 2005;493(1):15–20.
2. Brittain KR, Peet SM, Castleden CM. Stroke and incontinence. Stroke. 1998;29(2):524–8.
3. Brittain KR, Perry SI, Peet SM, Shaw C, Dallosso H, Assassa RP, et al. Prevalence and impact of urinary symptoms among community-dwelling stroke survivors. Stroke. 2000;31(4):886–91.
4. Rotar M, Blagus R, Jeromel M, Skrbec M, Trsinar B, Vodusek DB. Stroke patients who regain urinary continence in the first week after acute first-ever stroke have better prognosis than patients with persistent lower urinary tract dysfunction. Neurourol Urodyn. 2011;30(7): 1315–8.
5. Kuptniratsaikul V, Kovindha A, Suethanapornkul S, Manimmanakorn N, Archongka Y. Complications during the rehabilitation period in Thai patients with stroke: a multicenter prospective study. Am J Phys Med Rehabil. 2009;88(2):92–9.
6. Kim TG, Yoo KH, Jeon SH, Lee HL, Chang SG. Effect of dominant hemispheric stroke on detrusor function in patients with lower urinary tract symptoms. Int J Urol. 2010;17(7):656–60.
7. Patel M, Coshall C, Rudd AG, Wolfe CD. Natural history and effects on 2-year outcomes of urinary incontinence after strokes. Stroke. 2011;32:122–7.
8. Moisey CU, Rees RW. Results of transurethral resection of prostate in patients with cerebrovascular disease. Br J Urol. 1978;50(7):539–41.
9. Chua K. Urinary incontinence after traumatic brain injury: incidence outcomes and correlates. Brain Inj. 2003;17(6):469–78.
10. Su Y, Zhang X, Zeng J, Pei Z, Cheung RT, Zhou QP, et al. New-onset constipation at acute stage after first stroke: incidence, risk factors, and impact on the stroke outcome. Stroke. 2009;40:1304–9.
11. Paris G, Gourcerol G, Leroi AM. Management of neurogenic bowel dysfunction. Eur J Phys Rehabil Med. 2011;47(4):661–76.
12. Camara-Lemarroy CR, Ibarra-Yruegas BE, Gongora-Rivera F. Gastrointestinal complications after ischemic stroke. J Neurol Sci. 2014;346(1–2):20–5.
13. Dusenbury W, Johansen PP, Mosack V, Steinke EE. Determinants of sexual function and dysfunction in men and women with stroke: a systematic review. Int J Clin Pract. 2017;71(7) https://doi.org/10.1111/ijcp.12969.
14. Finazzi Agrò E, Musco S, D' Amico A. Lower urinary tract dysfunction following traumatic brain injury. Urodinamica. 2007;17(3):154–5.

15. Giannantoni E, Silvestro D, Siracusano S, et al. Urologic dysfunction and neurologic outcome in coma survivors after severe traumatic brain injury in the postacute and chronic phase. Arch Phys Med Rehabil. 2011;92(7):1134–8.
16. Olsen AB, Hetz RA, Xue H, Aroom KR, Bhattarai D, Johnson E, Bedi S, Cox CS Jr, Uray K. Effects of traumatic brain injury on intestinal contractility. Neurogastroenterol Motil. 2013;25(7):593–e463.
17. Sander AM, Maestas KL, Pappadis MR, et al. Multicenter study of sexual functioning in spouses/partners of persons with traumatic brain injury. Arch Phys Med Rehabil. 2016;97(5):753–9.
18. Turner D, Schottle D, Krueger R, Briken P. Sexual behavior and its correlates after traumatic brain injury. Curr Opin Psychiatry. 2015;28(2):180–7.
19. Sakakibara R, Kanda T, Sekido T, et al. Mechanism of bladder dysfunction in idiopathic normal pressure hydrocephalus. Neurourol Urodyn. 2008;27:507–10.
20. Campos-Juanatey F, Gutierrez-Banos JL, Portillo-Martin JA, et al. Assessment of the urodynamic diagnosis in patients with urinary incontinence associated with normal pressure hydrocephalus. Neurourol Urodyn. 2015;34:465.
21. Krzastek SC, Robinson SP, Young HF, Klausner AP. Improvement in lower urinary tract symptoms across multiple domains following ventriculoperitoneal shunting for idiopathic normal pressure hydrocephalus. Neurourol Urodyn. 2017;36(8):2056–63. https://doi.org/10.1002/nau.23235.
22. Ezzat AAM, Soliman MAR, Hasanain AA, et al. Migration of the distal catheter of ventriculoperitoneal shunts in pediatric age group: case series. World Neurosurg. 2018;119:e131–7. https://doi.org/10.1016/j.wneu.2018.07.073.
23. Richards CL, Malouin F. Cerebral palsy: definition, assessment and rehabilitation. Handb Clin Neurol. 2013;111:183–95.
24. Samiijn B, Vanlaecke E. Lower urinary tract symptoms and urodynamic findings in children and adults with cerebral palsy: a systematic review. Neurourol Urodyn. 2017;36(3):541–9.
25. Samijn B. Risk factors for daytime or combined incontinence in children with cerebral palsy. J Urol. 2017;198:937.
26. Wright AJ, Fletcher O, Scrutton D, Baird G. Bladder and bowel continence in bilateral cerebral palsy: a population study. J Pediatr Urol. 2016;12(6):383.
27. Wiegerink DJHG, Roebroeck ME, Donkervoort M, et al. Social, intimate and sexual relationships of adolescents with cerebral palsy compared with able-bodied age-mates. J Rehabil Med. 2008;40(2):112–8.
28. Okorji LM, Oberlin D. Lower urinary tract symptoms secondary to mass lesion of the brain: a case report and review of the literature. Urol Case Rep. 2016;8:7–8.
29. Sakakibara R, Shinotoh H, Uchiyama T, Sakuma M, Kashiwado M, Yoshiyama M, et al. Questionnaire-based assessment of pelvic organ dysfunction in Parkinson's disease. Auton Neurosci. 2001;92(1–2):76–85.
30. Araki I, Kuno S. Assessment of voiding dysfunction in Parkinson's disease by the international prostate symptom score. J Neurol Neurosurg Psychiatry. 2000;68(4):429–33.
31. Sakakibara R, Hattori T, Uchiyama T, Kita K, Asahina M, Suzuki A, et al. Urinary dysfunction and orthostatic hypotension in multiple system atrophy: which is the more common and earlier manifestation? J Neurol Neurosurg Psychiatry. 2000;68(1):65–9.
32. Ogawa T, Sakakibara R, Kuno S, Ishizuka O, Kitta T, Yoshimura N. Prevalence and treatment of LUTS in patients with Parkinson disease or multiple system atrophy. Nat Rev Urol. 2017;14(2):79–89.
33. Mishima T, Fukae J, Fujioka S, Inoue K, Tsuboi Y. The prevalence of constipation and irritable bowel syndrome in Parkinson's disease patients according to Rome III diagnostic criteria. J Park Dis. 2017;7(2):353–7.
34. Sakakibara R, Kishi M, Ogawa E, Tateno F, Uchiyama T, Yamamoto T, Yamanishi T. Bladder, bowel, and sexual dysfunction in Parkinson's disease. Parkinsons Dis. 2011;2011:924605.
35. Sung HY, Choi MG, Kim YI, Lee KS, Kim JS. Anorectal manometric dysfunctions in newly diagnosed, early-stage Parkinson's disease. J Clin Neurol. 2012;8:184–9.

36. Picillo M, Palladino R, Erro R, et al. The PRIAMO study: active sexual life is associated with better motor and non-motor outcomes in men with early Parkinson's disease. Eur J Neurol. 2019; https://doi.org/10.1111/ene.13983.
37. Yamamoto T, Sakakibara R, Uchiyama T, et al. Pelvic organ dysfunction is more prevalent and severe in MSA-P compared to Parkinson's disease. Neurourol Urodyn. 2011;30(1):102–7.
38. Krimchansky B, Sazbon L, Heller L, et al. Bladder tone in post-traumatic vegetative state. Brain Inj. 1999;13:899–903.
39. Benecchi L, Caldera GL, Cavestro C, et al. Peculiarità cistomanometrica nel periodo post-comatoso. Urologia. 1996;63(Suppl)
40. Wyndaele JJ. Micturition in comatose patients. J Urol. 1986;135:1209–11.
41. Wyndaele J. Urodynamics in comatose patients. Neurourol Urodyn. 1990;9:43–52.

Management of the Central Nervous System Chronic Pelvic Pain

Marilena Gubbiotti and Antonella Giannantoni

Chronic pelvic pain (CPP) is a syndrome characterized by persistent pain lasting longer than 6 months, or recurrent and noncyclic episodes of abdominal/pelvic pain, hypersensitivity, or discomfort often associated with lower urinary tract, sexual, bowel, pelvic floor, or gynecological dysfunction and emotional consequences, often in the absence of an organic etiology [1].

Despite its high prevalence (CPP affects approximately 15–20% of women in the USA) and its negative impact on quality of life (QoL), little is known about the mechanisms underlying CPP [2]. The impact and burden of CPP to patients are enormous. CPP patients suffer from considerable morbidity throughout their lives, with a resulting, significant decrease in QoL which may affect also their partners. Chronic pelvic pain syndromes (CPPS) are multifactorial and multidisciplinary conditions [3] with possible sources of pain located in the urogynecological, gastrointestinal, and musculoskeletal tract, and/or in the nervous system (NS) [4].

CPP mechanisms may include ongoing acute *peripheral* pain mechanisms involving somatic or visceral tissue and/or chronic pain mechanisms, which especially involve the central nervous system (CNS; [5]). As of peripheral pain mechanisms, inflammatory pain results from the increased excitability of peripheral nociceptive sensory fibers produced by the action of inflammatory mediators. The release of substance P and other neurotransmitters, and gross mast cell activation, results in neurogenic inflammation [6]. This excitatory effect, in turn, is a result of the altered activity of ion channels within affected sensory fibers [7]. Activation of acute pain mechanisms by a nociceptive event may sensitize peripheral nociceptive

M. Gubbiotti (✉)
Department of Urology, San Donato Hospital, Arezzo, Italy

A. Giannantoni
Department of Medical and Surgical Sciences and Neurosciences, Functional and Surgical Urology Unit, University of Siena, Siena, Italy
e-mail: antonella.giannantoni@unisi.it

© Springer Nature Switzerland AG 2020
G. Lamberti et al. (eds.), *Suprapontine Lesions and Neurogenic Pelvic Dysfunctions*, Urodynamics, Neurourology and Pelvic Floor Dysfunctions,
https://doi.org/10.1007/978-3-030-29775-6_6

afferents, magnifying the afferent signalling [8, 9]. When pain becomes long-lasting and the afferent signaling from the periphery to CNS continues to be over-functioning, a *central sensitization* (CS) can occur, although the initial injury can be completely disappeared [10]. The peripheral sensitization is a local event, while CS is a central phenomenon of the NS with the enhanced responsiveness of the central neurons to input from unimodal and polymodal receptors and there is no ongoing nociceptive stimulation from the periphery [11]. This central hypersensitivity could clarify the presence of chronic pain in the absence of a recognized peripheral pathology [12]. A continuous pain signal from the pelvis may result in a dysfunctional CNS response know as central pain amplification [13]. The "widespread pain" may be independent of pain severity and could imply a restructuring of pain processing at the level of the brain.

6.1   Neuroimaging

The mechanisms contributing to pain amplification and chronicity are heterogeneous and likely occur at various levels of the NS. Tests that look at brain structure and function (e.g., neuroimaging studies) can help diagnosis and define certain pain conditions. Types of neuroimaging tests include computed tomography, magnetic resonance imaging (MRI), and positron-emission tomography. In pelvic pain conditions, functional MRIs may be used to confirm symptoms in patients suffering from painful conditions. Neuroimaging techniques using MRI have allowed the detailed description of the brain in patients with CPP. Alterations in structural brain regions and regional connectivity are associated with pain perception and modulation in the affected patients. A decrease in gray matter density/volume in the thalamus, cingulate cortex, insular cortex, and cerebellum has been demonstrated in patients with chronic pain syndromes [2]. Moreover, alterations in regional brain morphology have been hypothesized to be responsible not only for the development and/or maintenance of pain but also for other common characteristics, such as mood disorders and cognitive impairment [14]. Kutch et al. demonstrated an increasing gray matter volume from the localized to intermediate and to widespread pain groups within several sensorimotor areas; moreover, the functional interaction between 37 pairs of brain regions increased significantly in CPP patients with widespread pain as compared to localized type [15].

6.2   Patient Assessment: Symptoms and Signs in Chronic Pelvic Pain

The diagnosis of CPP is solely symptomatic and comes from the history of pain perceived in the region of the pelvis, in the absence of other pathologies. Medical history and physical examination are the most important steps to understand better the patient's perception of his/her pain. Examination should provide for specific questions about duration, perception, and modality of pain [16]. The onset of symptoms may be either gradual or rapid. Therefore, the diagnosis is based on the exclusion of confusable illness and on the presence of specific combination of symptoms and signs [17].

Common bladder symptoms of CPP include increased daytime and nighttime urinary frequency, urgency, bladder hypersensitivity, bladder discomfort, and bladder pain: these symptoms are collectively called hypersensitive bladder syndrome [18]. According to the ESSIC Guidelines [17], urinary symptoms should be investigated by urinalyses and urine cultures, PSA in males >40 years, uroflowmetry, post-void residual urinary volume by ultrasound scanning, cystoscopy, and bladder wall biopsy.

Questionnaires are validated instruments to assess urinary and sexual dysfunction, pain, disability, fatigue, mood, and sleep disorders [19]. The most frequently used questionnaire for the evaluation of pain, urinary symptoms, and QoL is the O'Leary/Sant (ICSI and ICPI).

In order to classify patients with CPP a 6-point clinical phenotyping system UPOINT (urinary, psychosocial, organ-specific, infection, neurologic/systemic, tenderness) has been clinically validated. Each domain is clinically defined and associated with specific therapy [20].

6.3   Treatment

Few well-designed, randomized controlled trials have been conducted until now on different treatment modalities, and this still precludes the development of evidence-based management strategies. Moreover, the majority of pharmacological agents used to treat patients with CPP are still off label [21]. To date, there is general agreement on the use of some agents (orally or intravesically administered) as indicated by the EAU guidelines on chronic pelvic pain [22] and the AUA Guidelines [23]. Severe CPP is difficult to treat and it often requires the use of antidepressants and anticonvulsants due to their additional analgesic properties. Benefit from medications used to control neuropathic pain may provide indirect evidence of the intrinsic nature of chronic pain [24]. The key point includes tailoring therapy to each patient on the basis of localization, severity, frequency, and duration of pain episodes. Thus, phenotyping of the disease condition based on symptom classification such as the UPOINT system is important for the selection of appropriate treatments in individual patients [25].

The management of CPP required a multifaceted approach of the pharmacological therapy due to the multiple levels in the nervous system which act in the mechanism of action of pain. In order to control central sensitization in patients affected by chronic pelvic pain, the EAU Guidelines recommended the following approach:

6.3.1   First-Line Agents

6.3.1.1 Antidepressants
Tricyclic antidepressants (TCA) are a treatment option frequently used for CPP. They act to increase the levels of norepinephrine and serotonin via reuptake

inhibition. Higher levels of norepinephrine and serotonin seem to decrease pain sensitivity [26]. There are research evidences that showed the role of amitriptyline in pain control as demonstrated by the study of van Opoven et al. [27]. Foster et al. demonstrated also a great effect of amitriptyline (increasing doses from 10 to 75 mg/day for 12 weeks) in reducing ICSI scores and urinary frequency [28]. Unfortunately, amitriptyline is associated with high rates of anticholinergic side effects, as dry mouth, dizziness, sedation, and constipation that can cause its early discontinuation [29].

Secondary amine tricyclics (e.g., nortriptyline and desipramine) have less anticholinergic side effects, and thus they seem to be preferable in terms of tolerability, although they show a lower effect in reducing painful symptoms [30].

Selective serotonin reuptake inhibitors (SSRI) such as paroxetine or fluoxetine can be used as antipsychotics. Indeed, they are normally used for agitation and delirium but their role in the management of chronic pain is unclear [31].

Other antidepressants (serotonin norepinephrine reuptake inhibitors—SNRI), such as duloxetine or venlafaxine, may have an analgesic effect by centrally increasing the norepinephrine levels. These drugs are usually well tolerated with few side effects but the available data on their efficacy are still very limited. Studies have been performed predominantly in patients with peripheral neuropathic pain and only few data are available for central pain [31].

Few data are actually available about the use of trazodone (serotonin-2 antagonist/reuptake inhibitor); the real benefit of this therapy is that it does not induce sexual dysfunction.

TCAs should be used with caution along with other drugs due to the possible emergence of the serotonin syndrome.

6.3.1.2 Membrane Stabilizers/Anticonvulsants

The mechanism of action of gabapentin and pregabalin is the calcium channel block, decreasing the reuptake of glutamate, substance P, and norepinephrine. These drugs are membrane stabilizers due their effect to reduce the hyperexcitability of nerves centrally and peripherally. Research evidences regarding the efficacy of anticonvulsants in CPP are limited. Sator-Katzenschlager et al. showed in their study that gabapentin improves pain symptoms compared to amitriptyline, with less side effects [32].

6.3.2   Second-Line Agents

6.3.2.1 Opioids

There are no data supporting the use of opioids in patients with CPP [33]. Opioids act directly to the μ or δ receptors that are found in both the central and peripheral nervous systems. Actually, opioids are the second-line therapy of moderate and severe pain. Their use in the treatment of chronic and nonmalignant pain in the long term is strongly discouraged and considered as the last chance. Recent research evidences have highlighted the opioid-induced hyperalgesia effect, a condition where paradoxically patients assuming opioids become more sensitive to certain painful stimuli [34]. Chronic opioid therapy is associated with multiple side effects such as immunosuppression, androgen deficiency (with lowered sex hormones), constipation, and depression [35]. The risk for their misuse must be constantly evaluated.

Other options other than traditional opioid treatment are opioids with a dual-acting components in order to increase their analgesic effect. Tapentadol, for example, is a centrally acting μ-opioid agonist with a norepinephrine reuptake inhibition. This dual mechanism allows for a greater use of the drug with less side effects [36].

6.3.2.2 Tramadol

The analgesic effect of tramadol includes weak μ-opioid agonist activity and weak reuptake inhibition of norepinephrine and serotonin. The Food and Drug Administration (FDA) recently issued a warning indicating that tramadol should be used with caution in older patients with seizures or on drugs that cause serotonin syndrome [37].

6.3.3 Third-Line Agents

6.3.3.1 Cannabinoids

Their features are the low side effect profile and poor risk of drug interactions. Targets for treatment are the two G-protein cannabinoid receptors: cannabinoid 1 (CB1r) and cannabinoid 2 (CB2r) which are strictly involved in pain modulation. Cannabinoid ligands are also important components in nociception of pain. While CB1r is widely expressed in the brain, CB2r is commonly found in the immune system (microglia and monocytes; [38]). Localization of CB1r to neuronal terminals strongly suggests that it plays important roles in regulating synaptic function. CB2r overexpression in microglia and central neurons has been demonstrated in mice with a consequent, genetically mediated improvement in CB2 signaling; conversely, the deletion of CB2r resulted in enhanced neuro-inflammatory response after sciatic nerve transection [39]. No data are available on the efficacy of cannabinoids in the treatment of CPP; few evidences about their use in other chronic pain conditions demonstrated variable effectiveness.

6.3.4 Fourth-Line Agents

6.3.4.1 Antipsychotics

Nix et al. in their meta-analysis on the analgesic potency of antipsychotics showed that only 10 out of 15 studies with a higher statistical power described a possible analgesic effect. None of the studies identified could differentiate between the effect of analgesia and sedation of the drug used. Evidences regarding the efficacy in pain reduction are inadequate and before using this drug as an add-on therapy it is necessary to consider adverse effects.

6.3.4.2 Other Anticonvulsant Agents

Topiramate: Few data are present about anticonvulsant in CPP. Muehlbacher et al. demonstrated the beneficial effects (in terms of pain and health-related quality of life) of topiramate in patients with chronic low back pain [40].

6.3.5   Emerging Therapies

6.3.5.1 Toxins

More recently, botulinum toxin (BTX) has also been used in pain-related disorders (on-label chronic migraine or off-label, such as neuropathic pain or lower back pain). Although BTX was initially considered to alleviate pain through a simple muscle relaxation, recent studies showed that the mechanism of action of BTX in pain relief is more complex [41]. A possible explanation for BTX-modulating pain is represented by its retrograde axonal transport to the CNS. It has been observed that, in addition to local uptake in the synaptic terminal, a distinct secondary uptake pathway results in retrograde transport of the fully active neurotoxin at distal sites. This retrograde axonal transport is followed by a process of cell-to-cell transfer (named trans-cytosis) by which the neurotoxin may gain access to second-order neurons in the CNS [42].

In CCI-exposed mice, BTX-A reduced the following: the number of astrocytes, the percentage of active astrocytes, and the activation of microglia in neuropathic animals after chronic morphine treatment, and it modulates the immune response through a TLR2-dependent pathway in macrophages [43].

6.3.6   Combination Therapies

6.3.6.1 Palmitoylethanolamide

The beginning and the maintenance of neuropathic pain include the link between neurons and nonneuronal immunocompetent cells (mast cells and microglia) with a cascade of pro- and anti-inflammatory cytokines: this concept introduces an important innovation in pain management. Palmitoylethanolamide (PEA) is a member of the N-acylethanolamine family of fatty acid amide signaling molecules, with antiallodynic and antihyperalgesic properties. PEA acts by downmodulating pro-inflammatory mediator release from mast cells and reducing mast cell and microglial cell activation [44]. At the molecular level, PEA is a peroxisome proliferator-activated receptor alpha (PPAR-α) ligand that performs anti-inflammatory, analgesic, and neuroprotective actions [45]. Few clinical studies demonstrated the efficacy and tolerability of ultramicronized PEA (um-PEA) in the treatment of multiple syndromes associated with chronic pain, poorly responsive to conventional pharmacological regimens, as add-on therapy [46]. Actually, no data are present regarding the use of PEA in CPP.

References

1. Nickel JC, Shoskes DA, Wagenlehner FH. Management of chronic prostatitis/chronic pelvic pain syndrome (CP/CPPS): the studies, the evidence, and the impact. World J Urol. 2013;31:747–53.
2. As-Sanie S, Harris RE, Napadow V, Kim J, Neshewat G, Kairys A, Williams D, Clauw DJ, Schmidt-Wilcke T. Changes in regional gray matter volume in women with chronic pelvic pain: a voxel based morphometry study. Pain. 2012;153:1006–14.
3. Doggweiler R, Whitmore KE, Meijlink JM, Drake MJ, Frawley H, Nordling J, Hanno P, Fraser MO, Homma Y, Garrido G, Gomes MJ, Elneil S, van de Merwe JP, Lin ATL, Tomoe H. A standard for terminology in chronic pelvic pain syndromes: a report from the chronic pelvic pain working group of the international continence society. Neurourol Urodyn. 2017;36(4):984–1008.
4. Apte G, Nelson P, Brismee JM, Dedrick G, Justiz R 3rd, Sizer PS Jr. Chronic female pelvic pain-Part 1: clinical pathoanatomy and examination of the pelvic region. Pain Pract. 2012;12:88–110.
5. Linley JE, Rose K, Ooi L, Gamper N. Understanding inflammatory pain: ion channels contributing to acute and chronic nociception. Pflugers Arch. 2010;459:657–69.
6. Zieglgansberger W, Berthele A, Tolle TR. Understanding neuropathic pain. CNS Spectr. 2005;10(4):298–308.
7. McMahon SB, Dmitrieva N, Koltzenburg M. Visceral pain. Br J Anaesth. 1995;75(2):132–44.
8. Wesselmann U, Baranowski AP, Borjesson M, Curran NC, Czakanski PP, Giamberardino MA, Ness TJ, Robbins MT, Traub RJ. Emerging therapies and novel approaches to visceral pain. Drug Discov Today Ther Strateg. 2009;6:89–95.
9. Giamberardino MA, Costantini R, Affaitati G, Fabrizio A, Lapenna D, Tafuri E, Mezzetti A. Viscero-visceral hyperalgesia: characterization in different clinical models. Pain. 2010;151:307–22.
10. Nijs J, Goubert D, Ickmans K. Recognition and treatment of central sensitization in chronic pain patients: not limited to specialized care. J Orthop Sports Phys Ther. 2016;46(12):1024–8.
11. Janicki TI. Chronic pelvic pain as a form of complex regional pain syndrome. Clin Obstet Gynecol. 2003;46:797–803.
12. As-Sanie S, Harris RE, Napadow V, Kim J, Neshewat G, Kairys A, Williams D, Clauw DJ, Schmidt-Wilcke T. Changes in regional gray matter volume in women with chronic pelvic pain: a voxel-based morphometry study. Pain. 2012;153:1006–14.
13. Giesecke T, Gracely RH, Grant MA, Nachemson A, Petzke F, Williams DA, Clauw DJ. Evidence of augmented central pain processing in idiopathic chronic low back pain. Arthritis Rheum. 2004;50(2):613–23.
14. Du MY, Wu QZ, Yue Q, Li J, Liao Y, Kuang WH, Huang XQ, Chan RC, Mechelli A, Gong QY. Voxelwise meta-analysis of gray matter reduction in major depressive disorder. Prog Neuro-Psychopharmacol Biol Psychiatry. 2012;36(1):11–6.
15. Kutch JJ, Ichesco E, Hampson JP, et al. Brain signature and functional impact of centralized pain: a multidisciplinary approach to the study of chronic pelvic pain (MAPP) network study. Pain. 2017;158(10):1979–91.
16. Abrams P, Cardozo L, Fall M, et al. The standardisation of terminology in lower urinary tract function: report from the standardisation sub-committee of the international continence society. Urology. 2003;61:37–49.
17. van de Merwe JP, Nordling J, Bouchelouche P, Bouchelouche K, Cervigni M, Daha LK, Elneil S, Fall M, Hohlbrugger G, Irwin P, Mortensen S, van Ophoven A, Osborne JL, Peeker R, Richter B, Riedl C, Sairanen J, Tinzl M, Wyndaele JJ, et al. Diagnostic criteria, classification, and nomenclature for painful bladder syndrome/interstitial cystitis: an ESSIC proposal. Eur Urol. 2008;53(1):60–7.

18. Homma Y, Ueda T, Tomoe H, Lin AT, Kuo HC, Lee MH, Lee JG, Kim DY, Lee KS, Interstitial cystitis guideline committee. Clinical guidelines for interstitial cystitis and hypersensitive bladder syndrome. Int J Urol. 2009;16:597–615.
19. Sutcliffe S, Gallop R, Henry Lai HH, Andriole GL, Bradley CS, Chelimsky G, Chelimsky T, Quentin Clemens J, Colditz GA, Erickson B, Griffith JW, Kim J, Krieger JN, Labus J, Naliboff BD, Rodriguez LV, Sutherland SE, Taple BJ, Landis JR. "Multidisciplinary approach to the study of chronic pelvic pain" (MAPP) research network. BJU Int. 2019;
20. Shoskes DA, Curtis Nickel J, Kattan MW. Phenotypically directed multimodal therapy for chronic prostatitis/chronic pelvic pain syndrome: a prospective study using UPOINT. Urology. 2010;10:1249–53.
21. Giannantoni A, Gubbiotti M, Yoshimura N, Andersson KE. Pharmacologic goals in interstitial cystitis/bladder pain syndrome. In: Hanno P, Nordling J, Wyndaele JJ, Staskin D, Wein A, editors. Bladder pain syndrome - an evolution. Berlin: Springer-Verlag; 2017. p. 87–94.
22. Engeler DS, Baranowski AP, Dinis-Oliveira P, Elneil S, Hughes J, Messelink EJ, van Ophoven A, Williams AC, European Association of Urology. The 2013 EAU guidelines on chronic pelvic pain: is management of chronic pelvic pain a habit, a philosophy, or a science? 10 years of development. Eur Urol. 2013;64:431–9.
23. Hanno PM, Burks DA, Clemens JQ, Dmochowski RR, Erickson D, Fitzgerald MP, Forrest JB, Gordon B, Gray M, Mayer RD, Newman D, Nyberg L Jr, Payne CK, Wesselmann U, Faraday MM, Interstitial Cystitis Guidelines Panel of the American Urological Association Education and Research, Inc. AUA guideline for the diagnosis and treatment of interstitial cystitis/bladder pain syndrome. J Urol. 2011;185:2162–70.
24. Siden HB, Carleton BC, Oberlander TF. Physician variability in treating pain and irritability of unknown origin in children with severe neurological impairment. Pain Res Manag. 2013;18(5):243–8.
25. Fall M, Logadottir Y, Peeker R. Interstitial cystitis is bladder pain syndrome with Hunner's lesion. Int J Urol. 2014;21(Suppl 1):79–82.
26. Tamano R, Ishida M, Asaki T. Effect of spinal monoaminergic neuronal system dysfunction on pain threshold in rats, and the analgesic effect of serotonin and norepinephrine reuptake inhibitors. Neurosci Lett. 2016;615:78–82.
27. van Ophoven A, Pokupic S, Heinecke A, Hertle L. A prospective, randomized, placebo controlled, double-blind study of amitriptyline for the treatment of interstitial cystitis. J Urol. 2004;172:533–6.
28. Foster HE, Hanno PM, Nickel JC, et al. Effect of amitriptyline on symptoms in treatment naive patients with interstitial cystitis/painful bladder syndrome. J Urol. 2010;183:1853–8.
29. An update on the drug treatment of neuropathic pain. Part 1: antidepressants. Drug Ther Bull. 2012;50:114–7.
30. Godfrey RG. A guide to the understanding and use of tricyclic antidepressant in the overall management of fibromyalgia and other chronic pain syndromes. Arch Intern Med. 1996;156:1047–52.
31. Hauer J, Houtrow AJ. Pain assessment and treatment in children with significant impairment of the central nervous system. Pediatrics. 2017;139(6):e20171002.
32. Sator-Katzenschlager SM, Scharbert G, Kress HG, Frickey N, Ellend A, Gleiss A, Kozek-Langenecker SA. Chronic pelvic pain treated with gabapentin and amitriptyline: a randomized controlled pilot study. Wien Klin Wochenschr. 2005;117:761–8.
33. Baranowski AP, Lee J, Price C, et al. Pelvic pain: a pathway for care developed for both men and women by the British pain society. Br J Anaesth. 2014;112(3):452–9.
34. Lee M, Silverman SM, Hansen H, Patel VB, Manchikanti L. A comprehensive review of opioid-induced hyperalgesia. Pain Physician. 2011;14:145–61.
35. Baber Z, Erdek MA. Failed back surgery syndrome: current perspectives. J Pain Res. 2016;9:979–87.
36. Carey ET, Till SR, As-Sanie S. Pharmacological management of chronic pelvic pain in women. Drugs. 2017;77(3):285–301.

37. Gardner JS, Blough D, Drinkard CR, Shatin D, Anderson G, Graham D, Alderfer R. Tramadol and seizures: a surveillance study in a managed care population. Pharmacotherapy. 2000;20(12):1423–31.
38. Howlett AC, Barth F, Bonner TI, Cabral G, Casellas P, Devane WA, Felder CC, Herkenham M, Mackie K, Martin BR, Mechoulam R, Pertwee RG. International Union of Pharmacology. XXVII. Classification of cannabinoid receptors. Pharmacol Rev. 2002;54:161–202.
39. Racz I, Nadal X, Alferink J, Baños JE, Rehnelt J, Martín M, Pintado B, Gutierrez-Adan A, Sanguino E, Manzanares J, Zimmer A, Maldonado R. Crucial role of CB(2) cannabinoid receptor in the regulation of central immune responses during neuropathic pain. J Neurosci. 2008;28:12125–35.
40. Muehlbacher M, Nickel MK, Kettler C, Tritt K, Lahmann C, Leiberich PK, Nickel C, Krawczyk J, Mitterlehner FO, Rother WK, Loew TH, Kaplan P. Topiramate in treatment of patients with chronic low back pain: a randomized, double-blind, placebo-controlled study. Clin J Pain. 2006;22:526–31.
41. Rivera Día RC, Lotero MAA, Suarez MVA, et al. Botulinum toxin for the treatment of chronic pain. Review of the evidence. Colomb J Anesthesiol. 2014;42:205–13.
42. Antonucci F, Rossi C, Gianfranceschi L, Rossetto O, Caleo M. Long-distance retrograde effects of botulinum neurotoxin A. J Neurosci. 2008;28(14):3689–96.
43. Vacca V, Marinelli S, Luvisetto S, Pavone F. Botulinum toxin A increases analgesic effects of morphine, counters development of morphine tolerance and modulates glia activation and μ opioid receptor expression in neuropathic mice. Brain Behav Immun. 2013;32:40–50.
44. Bettoni I, Comelli F, Colombo A, Bonfanti P, Costa B. Non-neuronal cell modulation relieves neuropathic pain: efficacy of the endogenous lipid palmitoylethanolamide. CNS Neurol Disord Drug Targets. 2013;12(1):34–44.
45. Alhouayek M, Muccioli GG. Harnessing the anti-inflammatory potential of palmitoylethanolamide. Drug Discov Today. 2014;19(10):1632–9.
46. Rao S, Song Y, Peddie F, Evans AM. Particle size reduction to the nanometer range: a promising approach to improve buccal absorption of poorly water-soluble drugs. Int J Nanomedicine. 2011;6:1245–51.

Management of Bowel Dysfunction in Patients with Central Nervous System Diseases

Gabriele Bazzocchi, Mimosa Balloni, Erica Poletti,
Roberta Manara, Paola Mongardi, Marica Vicchi,
Eugenia Fragalà, Elena Demertzis, Antonella Manzan,
and Humberto Cerrel Bazo

7.1 Introduction

Pathologies affecting the central nervous system (CNS), despite obvious differences in terms of lesion level, etiology, and comorbidities, involve alterations of digestive functions and, in particular, defecation disorders [1, 2]. This is not surprising when considering that the ability to control bladder and bowel emptying is the last function that the *Homo sapiens* "cub" learns: children start walking and talking before being able of avoiding micturition and defecation at inappropriate times and before diaper weaning. Acquiring this ability means having the encephalic and medullary centers of both the CNS and the autonomic nervous system (ANS) well organized in order to control the same muscle-fascial structures of the abdominal wall and of the pelvic floor, so that they can first be effective at holding urine, feces and gas, and then efficient at expelling them at chosen times thus ensuring a complete emptying. It is therefore clear how even minor injuries of nerve pathways and control centers can easily compromise this integrated and delicate visceral, pelvic, and perineal dynamic. The pathophysiological mechanisms underlying intestinal dysfunctions on a neurogenic basis are a mix of different elements:

G. Bazzocchi (✉) · M. Balloni · E. Poletti · R. Manara · P. Mongardi · M. Vicchi
NeuroGastroenterology and Intestinal Rehabilitation Unit, Montecatone Rehabilitation
Institute S.p.A., Imola (BO), Italy
e-mail: gabriele.bazzocchi@unibo.it; mimosa.balloni@montecatone.com;
erica.poletti@montecatone.com; roberta.manara@montecatone.com;
paola.mongardi@montecatone.com; marica.vicchi@montecatone.com

E. Fragalà
Department of Urology, Hospital G.B. Morgagni- L. Pierantoni of Forlí, Forlí-Cesena, Italy
e-mail: eugenia.fragala@montecatone.com

E. Demertzis · A. Manzan · H. Cerrel Bazo
Spinal Unit, Ospedale Riabilitativo di Alta Specializzazione S.p.A.,
Motta di Livenza (TV), Italy
e-mail: Elena.Demertzis@ospedalemotta.it; Antonella.Mazan@ospedalemotta.it

© Springer Nature Switzerland AG 2020
G. Lamberti et al. (eds.), *Suprapontine Lesions and Neurogenic Pelvic
Dysfunctions*, Urodynamics, Neurourology and Pelvic Floor Dysfunctions,
https://doi.org/10.1007/978-3-030-29775-6_7

reduced propulsion within the large intestine; abdominal-perineal dyssynergia due to deficiency and incoordination of pelvic floor muscles, associated with anorectal hyposensitivity; deficit of voluntary contraction of external anal sphincter; and abnormalities of internal sphincter reflex [3, 4]. There is ample literature that highlights how the management of intestinal evacuation is the most critical problem for people with CNS lesions once the acute phase is concluded, in terms of not only quality of life, but also morbidity and mortality [5, 6]. The term "neurogenic bowel" has been borrowed from bladder dysfunction, but there are many and significant differences between these two visceral disorders: while the level of the neurological lesion determines quite accurately which sequelae will be produced on bladder function (hyper-hypocompliant, hyper-hypoactive), this is not true for bowel, especially as regards intestinal motility. In the digestive tract wall lies a neuronal network which is comparable, in terms of number and complexity of cells and connections, to the brain, so much so that it is defined as a real "second brain," which allows the bowel to have its own peristalsis even if totally isolated from CNS and ANS [7]. The most relevant difference regards the type of content that is evacuated from the two organs: liquid from the bladder, from semiliquid to decidedly solid from the bowel. Moreover, the flow of urine is constant towards the bladder, while the filling of rectum (which is physiologically empty outside the defecatory event) shows great differences in terms of content volume and time for occurring. The fecal volume, in addition to water percentage, is determined by the presence of bacteria originating from the colon microflora [8]. The colon represents a real ecosystem with a concentration of microorganisms that has no equal in any other habitat on the planet Earth. Indeed, more than 1000 different bacterial groups live in the human intestine and form a biomass that can weigh up to 1.5 kg and has a huge (and mostly still unknown) metabolic activity: a sort of second liver made up of 100,000 billion prokaryotic cells [9]. It should be noted that the action of fibers and prebiotics is not due to a "mass" effect resulting from a recall of water produced by the polysaccharide molecules of which they are made up, but their action, which favors evacuation, derives from the fact that they constitute the main metabolic substrate for the colon microflora: the biomass grown this way constitutes 60–80% of the dry weight of the feces. It follows that the primary objective of intestinal rehabilitation, in a patient who has lost control and efficiency of evacuation mechanisms due to a CNS damage, is certainly to achieve defecation but not "di per sè," but as a way of rebalancing the ecosystem in the intestinal lumen [10]. Since it is often impossible to retrieve a physiological evacuation (as it is the case of micturition too), it is necessary to adopt methods for programming intestinal emptying, which could guarantee completeness and adequate times and, in the long run, are not detrimental to the anorectal region.

7.2   Objectives of Intestinal Rehabilitation in the Person with CNS Lesions

Contrary to what could be assumed, recovering a bowel evacuation as it was before the damaging event, that is spontaneous and following the perception of a "defecation need" signal, is not a primary rehabilitation goal: it is often impossible and it almost always exposes the patient to the risk of incontinence and incomplete emptying.

Instead, rehabilitation goals are the following:

1. To confine the defecation at the best time of the day according to the patient and the availability of assistance, with the certainty that the chosen method for this artificial and "programmed" evacuation is effective and the time does not exceed 60 min in total
2. To guarantee that the interval between two programmed defecations is free from unwanted evacuations, incontinence, or leakage
3. To avoid abdominal discomfort (swelling, abdominal distension, pain) and to prevent the occurrence of complications such as bleeding, hemorrhoidal disease, fissures, rectal mucosal prolapse, bowel dilatation, and fecal impaction in relation to the modality chosen for stimulation of defecation
4. To achieve the maximum independence/autonomy possible, together with safeguarding the best quality of life and dignity, while performing this delicate visceral function (use of the toilet/commode, freedom of evacuation in any toilet)
5. To guarantee a complete emptying avoiding accumulation and stagnation of fecal residues, an event that is not correlated to the frequency of evacuations and that cannot be excluded from a sense of well-being and satisfaction even for a long time
6. To contrast the translocation of normal commensal bacteria of the intestinal lumen (*E. coli*, Klebsiella, Enterobacteriaceae, *Streptococcus faecalis*, etc.) with consequent bladder contamination and episodes of colonization or urinary infection
7. Not to undermine the complex (and mostly still unknown) balance mechanisms of the intestinal microbiota avoiding excessive dietary manipulation, and use of antibiotics, stimulant, or irritating laxative drugs, while associating stimulation with the assumption of dietary supplements, osmotic laxatives, and prokinetic drugs which guarantee an optimal volume and consistency of the fecal mass

7.3   Tools for Assessment and Monitoring of Bowel Dysfunction

For a quantitative overview of bowel dysfunction, with particular regard to evacuation disorders, the following are useful tools of assessment and monitoring:

1. *Bowel diary*: A precise recording of weekly evacuations and an indispensable tool to register both the severity of alterations and the information on its possible causes, especially with information on evacuation modalities, i.e., spontaneous or stimulated and how stimulated [11].
2. *Classification of fecal consistency according to the Bristol Stool Form Scale* which identifies seven different types of feces: at the one end, scarce and hard lumps ("goatlike") with a score = 1, and on the other end completely liquid feces with a score = 7 [12, 13].
3. Graduation of *severity of intestinal dysfunction on a neurogenic basis obtained by calculating the neurogenic bowel dysfunction (NBD) score* proposed and vali-

dated by Klaus Krogh and colleagues and now universally used in studies of efficacy and clinical trials: The score identifies four classes of severity of constipation and incontinence in patients with spinal cord injuries by a 10-item questionnaire, including the impact on quality of life [14].

4. *Intestinal transit study*: It implies the ingestion of ten radiopaque markers for six consecutive days and the execution of a direct abdominal radiography on the seventh day, at the same time the markers were ingested. The total colonic transit time, expressed in hours, is calculated by counting the markers retained [15]. Since, as said, in SCI patients defecation must be scheduled, it is possible to match the execution of the final direct abdominal RX immediately after a defecation, with respect of the patient's intervals. It is thus possible to express a completeness evaluation of the evacuations occurred during the 7-day examination, in analogy to what is done with the post-void residual evaluation by bladder scanner after physiological urination or catheterization.

   This test should always be performed when a satisfactory balance of intestinal function is achieved. As a matter of fact, as already mentioned, it allows a precise indication of the degree of completeness of evacuations according to the methods implemented and, therefore, a full achievement of the rehabilitation objectives.

5. Interesting is the recently proposed method for evaluating segmental and total colon volumes which are defined on CT scans using dedicated software [16].

7.4 Care Devices

To set up an effective bowel management in a person with neurological lesions it is necessary to have, on the one hand, drugs and supplements that guarantee the formation and propulsion of colonic fecal contents, and, on the other hand, maneuvers with aids and devices that assist, or substitute for, the expulsive function.

The main types of *DRUGS and SUPPLEMENTS are listed below*:

- An osmotic laxative, such as macrogol 3550–4000, which can be taken continuously, so containing electrolytes in its composition, without the addition of sodium sulfate and with different formulations so as to adapt to any possible routes of administration (oral, PEG, transanal): The aim is to maintain the best consistency of the fecal mass, avoiding too harsh and "goatlike" stools, along with a correct nutrition and supplementation based on prebiotics, soluble fibers such as psyllium or glucomannans, and probiotics, both mono-strain and mixtures, in concentrations that guarantee an effective colonization [17–19].
- It is often necessary to obtain a complete bowel emptying, intensively and in a short time, as before a colonoscopy. The purpose is to solve a situation of massive coprostasis or to eliminate post-evacuation fecal residues that could accumulate even if patient shows regular defecation frequency following a correct treatment.
- This can be achieved in three ways:

- Assumption of a solution with a macrogol-based product, added to the lowest possible volume of water necessary for the same effect, due to the intaking difficulties often manifested by these patients, adaptable both to oral and PEG administration [20].
- Sodium phosphate-based laxative.
- One or more sessions of hydrocolon therapy: Through the use of a complex machine, peremptorily placed in hospitals or outpatient facilities and managed by specialized medical and nursing staff, it is possible to perform repeated retrograde colonic irrigations with large volumes of water (up to 50 L) alternating phases of loading with phases in which, through a special system of closed tubes, the content of the colorectal is unloaded into isolated containers. In some patients it is a useful recurrent aid to complement other daily measures in a variegated and multimodal bowel management [21, 22].
- Contact laxatives for continuous or cyclic use, such as sennosides A and B, bisacodyl, and picosulfate [23].
- Prokinetics and modulators of intestinal motility, such as prucalopride, linaclotide, trimebutine, levosulpiride, and intrastigmine [24, 25]. Positive effects are reported in some cases with erythromycin (3 mg/kg) and misoprostol [26, 27].
- Proctological gel and creams: Mesalazine-based and AC-based hyaluronic gels are useful as well as gels/ointments with a soothing effect and cortisone ointments.
- Nonabsorbable intestinal antibiotics, such as rifaximin, and other drugs, such as cholestyramine, intestinal antimuscarinics, and direct myolitics, such as mebeverine.

EVACUANTS, as suppositories of glycerine and bisacodyl, glycerine microclisms, sodium phosphate and hyperosmotic solutions, with or without sorbitol. Among them should also be included both anal digitation and actual manual maneuvers for extracting feces from the rectum, carried out by the patient or the caregiver.

DEVICES and various procedures for performing transanal irrigation (TAI) deserve a separate description:

- 60 mL Cone/catheter syringe connected to a 22–28–32 F rectal probe: Irrigation takes place with repeated introduction of water boluses with the possibility of varying the flow rate up to high values (30 mL/s).
- Rectoclysis with enema bag, after insertion of a rectal probe, which in some cases can be replaced by a 16 F Foley catheter, so as to ensure rectal anchoring and to prevent its expulsion during water entry: Irrigation should normally be performed by filling the bag with 2 L of saline, placed at least 150 cm above the anal canal. The flow must be fast enough to complete the irrigation in 7–10 min.
- Qufora® IrriSedo-PMC: It improves both previous methods as it allows the introduction of high volumes of water (even >1 L), as it happens with the rectoclysis, but without the inconvenience of preparing the system from above. At the same

time, it allows to regulate the flow, and its pressure, from minimum to very high values, as it happens with the cone/catheter syringe [28].

- Peristeen: It is the first device built on the concept of the "continence catheter," available for 12 years now [29, 30]. It allows the irrigation of the colon with 700–1000 mL of water that should be introduced in 3 min during which a "sealed chamber" condition of the large intestine is maintained, and, consequently, a mechanical stimulation on its walls, able to elicit intestinal peristalsis, is guaranteed. With "continence catheter" we define the rectal probes that allow inserting water in the colon, but at the same time are equipped with a balloon which, once insufflated, obstructs and blocks the patency of the anal canal. The sphincter continence is therefore guaranteed during the irrigation phase even in people with no voluntary contraction: neither the water introduced into the colon, even at positive pressure, nor the intestinal gas or liquid stool can in this way escape. The large intestine is thus transformed into a hollow, closed, and watertight organ, so the pressure exerted by the action of the pump on the water inside the container bag is transmitted inside the intestinal lumen. There is convincing evidence that even in the person with spinal cord injury, this intraluminal pressure increases by stretching the walls, induces the onset of peristaltic contractions with a propulsive effect that facilitates evacuation, and above all allows the physiological emptying of the whole left colon [31].

- Navina Smart: It is a device similar to the previous one as far as the concept and the TAI dynamics are concerned, but it is equipped with a computerized pump and selector, which make it possible to keep stable both air injection parameters in the rectal catheter balloon and volume and flow rate of irrigation water, once these have been established during training sessions with experienced operators. The procedure therefore does not undergo any small or large variations due to the force that the patient, or different caregivers, can exercise with manual pump devices. Furthermore, the rectal balloon volume, proposed by the system, is always the same, thus guaranteeing the stability of TAI parameters. In some cases, when using this device, tetraplegic patients with a partial use of upper limbs are able to perform the TAI procedure and consequently their bowel management independently, without any caregiver assistance.

- Qufora® IrriSedo-Care: It is a manual pump device, but unlike Peristeen the pressure, exerted directly on the irrigation water, is not constant, but undergoes variations, due to the frequency and force of the pump. It also differs from Peristeen and Navina Smart because the rectal catheter balloon is filled with water and not with air, thus guaranteeing a non-compressible volume and a more solid anchorage. This factor is sometimes the key to the efficacy of TAI, otherwise not obtainable.

7.5 "Step-by-Step" Approach to Bowel Management in the Person with CNS Lesions

On the basis of their long-standing experience, the authors suggest the following protocol:

7.5.1   First Step

- Specific dietary indications are given, together with recommendations for a correct daily caloric intake, to get at least 40% of the total daily calories from proteins, tending towards dietary fibers, which help maintain a proper hydration of the feces.
- Suspension of oral stimulant laxatives: their action makes it impossible to schedule any defecation timing.
- Scheduling of defecation every other day by means of evacuating measures, alone or in combination, depending on the effectiveness and tolerability evaluation performed by the team operators involved.
- Bowel diary included in medical records with monitoring of the percentage of failed evacuations and of hard and abnormal stools. In case of more than 20% of hard/abnormal stools or if management does not allow a satisfactory path towards rehabilitation goals, the second step is necessary.

7.5.2   Second Step

- Osmotic laxative intake, starting from a 10 to 30 g dose: The dose can be increased or decreased according to stool consistency; however the interval between dose modifications should not be less than 6 days.
- Osmotic laxatives, except in special cases, should always be associated with soluble fibers and probiotics intake. The aim is to obtain a type 4–5 stool consistency according to the Bristol Stool Form Scale in patients who anyway have a slowed-down transit despite defecation at programmed intervals.
- Evacuants can be associated with TAI with cone/catheter syringe or rectoclysis according to the effectiveness and tolerability evaluation performed by the team of operators involved.
- As regards manual assistance, the operators should assess whether various maneuvers can be partially helpful, if implemented to a very modest extent, appropriate for general status of the patient, or they actually constitute the fundamental element of a successful bowel care. If this is the case, this will constitute a precise indication of introduction of TAI with "positive-pressure" devices.
- As regards oral stimulant laxatives, their use can be proposed, since it is considered useful at certain times, to overcome some temporary problems, in preparation to particular diagnostic programs. In this case too, the necessity of their continuous use will constitute a precise indication to the introduction of TAI with "positive-pressure" devices.

7.5.3   Third Step: Adoption of TAI with "Positive-Pressure" Devices

As previously seen, Qufora® IrriSedo-PMC and Care, Peristeen, and Navina Smart are equipped with this feature.

The decision to base bowel management on the use of these devices can result from the following situations:

- After 2 weeks of continuous application of second step indications, intestinal emptying difficulties are not resolved and rehabilitation goals are not satisfactorily achieved.
- The constant and important use of manual maneuvers is mandatory; otherwise bowel management is not successful.
- Without the use of oral stimulant laxatives, a defecation schedule with no failures is not guaranteed.
- According to the patient's point of view and the evaluation of the team of operators, the trend towards objectives is satisfactory, but the study of the intestinal transit with markers shows a remarkable retention and therefore incompleteness of the planned evacuations.
- The neurogenic bowel dysfunction score does not fall below 10 or the Bristol Stool Form Scale score remains predominantly >6 (too fluid) or <3 (too hard).
- It is clear that TAI would allow performing bowel emptying on the toilet/commode, while every other mode should be carried out at the bed. It should therefore be adopted if this factor constitutes a real advantage included in the final rehabilitation project of the patient.
- Same thing if TAI performed with "positive-pressure" devices is preferred by the patient beyond any consideration of the effectiveness of the treatment with evacuants and/or TAI with syringe, rectoclysis with or without rectal probe: In this case too, the evaluation of opportunity/appropriateness of its adoption will be evaluated within the framework of the definitive project.

As regards the choice of the device, there are no comparative studies, no guidelines, and no simple lines of conduct to follow: the operators' experience is fundamental together with verification on the field of the tolerability/effectiveness ratio, taking into account the many variables of intestinal expulsive dynamics in relation to the pathology and having a complete knowledge of the functioning of the different devices. Certainly, to date, the greatest experience reported in literature is the prerogative of the Peristeen, so it seems logical to the authors to consider it, in the absence of other precise clinical considerations, as a first-choice device. In the near future there will be studies that will more precisely define the indications of the various devices in relation to their specific differences in construction and operation [32, 33].

Acknowledgments The authors are indebted to Dr. Cecilia Baroncini, Scientific Office of the Montecatone Rehabilitation Institute, for the secretarial assistance.

References

1. Krogh K, Christensen P. Neurogenic colorectal and pelvic floor dysfunction. Best Pract Res Clin Gastroenterol. 2009;23:531–43.
2. Bazzocchi G, Schuijt C, Pederzini R, Menarini M. Bowel dysfunction in spinal cord injury patients: pathophysiology and management. Pelviperineology. 2007;26:84–7.

3. Valles M, Mearin F. Pathophysiology of bowel dysfunction in patients with motor incomplete spinal cord injury: comparison with patients with motor complete spinal cord injury. Dis Colon Rectum. 2009;52:1589–97.
4. Salvioli B, Bazzocchi G, Barbara G, Stanghellini V, Cremon C, Menarini M, Corinaldesi R, De Giorgio R. Sigmoid compliance and visceral perception in spinal cord injury patients. Eur J Gastroenterol Hepatol. 2012;24:340–5.
5. Burns AS, St-Germain D, Connolly M, Delparte JJ, Guindon A, Hitzig SL, Craven BC. Phenomenological study of neurogenic bowel from the perspective of individuals living with spinal cord injury. Arch Phys Med Rehabil. 2015;96:49–55.
6. Patel DP, Elliott SP, Stoffel JT, Brant WO, Hotaling JM, Myers JB. Patient reported outcomes measures in neurogenic bladder and bowel: a systematic review of the current literature. Neurourol Urodyn. 2016;35:8–14.
7. Costa M, Wiklendt L, Simpson P, Spencer NJ, Brookes SJ, Dinning PG. Neuromechanical factors involved in the formation and propulsion of fecal pellets in the guinea-pig colon. Neurogastroenterol Motil. 2015;10:1466–77.
8. Vandeputte D, Falony G, Vieira-Silva S, Tito RY, Joossens M, Raes J. Stool consistency is strongly associated with gut microbiota richness and composition, enterotypes and bacterial growth rates. Gut. 2016;65:57–62.
9. Bengmark S. Ecological control of the gastrointestinal tract. The role of probiotic flora. Gut. 1998;42:2–7.
10. Quigley EMM. The enteric microbiota in the pathogenesis and management of constipation. Best Pract Res Clin Gastroenterol. 2011;25:119–26.
11. Juul T, Bazzocchi G, Coggrave M, Johannesen IL, Hansen RBM, Thiyagaraian C, Poletti E, Krogh K, Christensen P. Reliability of the international spinal cord injury bowel function basic and extended data sets. Spinal Cord. 2011;49:886–92.
12. Blake MR, Raker JM, Whelan K. Validity and reliability of the Bristol stool form scale in healthy adults and patients with diarrhea-predominant irritable bowel syndrome. Aliment Pharmacol Ther. 2016;44:693–703.
13. Chumpitazi BP, Self MM, Czyzewski DI, Cejka S, Swank PR, Shulman RJ. Bristol Stool Form Scale reliability and agreement decreases when determining Rome III stool form designation. Neurogastroenterol Motil. 2016;28:443–8.
14. Krogh K, Christensen P, Sabroe S, Laurberg S. Neurogenic bowel dysfunction score. Spinal Cord. 2006;44:625–31.
15. Abrahamsson H, Antov S. Accuracy in assessment of colonic transit time with particles: how many markers should be used? Neurogastroenterol Motil. 2010;22:1164–9.
16. Knudsen K, Fedorova TD, Bekker AC, Iversen P, Ostergaard K, Krogh K, Borghammer P. Objective colonic dysfunction is far more prevalent than subjective constipation in Parkinson's disease: a colon transit and volume study. J Park Dis. 2017;7:359–67.
17. Corazziari E, Badiali D, Bazzocchi G, Bassotti G, Roselli P, Mastropaolo G, Lucà MG, Galeazzi R, Peruzzi E. Long term efficacy, safety, and tolerability of low daily doses of isosmotic polyethylene glycol electrolyte balanced solution (PMF-100) in the treatment of functional chronic constipation. Gut. 2000;46:522–6.
18. Bazzocchi G. Polyethylene glycol solution in subgroups of chronic constipation patients: experience in obstructed defaecation. Ital J Gastroenterol Hepatol. 1999;31(Suppl.3):S257–9.
19. Bazzocchi G, Giussani C, Brigidi P, Turroni S. Effect of a symbiotic preparation on symptoms, stool consistency, intestinal transit time and gut microbiota in patients with severe functional constipation: a double blind, controlled trial. Tech Coloproctol. 2014;18:945–53.
20. DeMicco MP, Clayton LB, Pilot J, Epstein MS, NOCT Study Group. Novel 1 L polyethylene glycol-based bowel preparation NER 1006 for overall and right-sided colon cleansing: a randomized controlled phase 3 trial versus trisulfate. Gastrointest Endosc. 2018;87:677–88.
21. Bazzocchi G, Giuberti R. Irrigation, lavage, colonic hydrotherapy: from beauty center to clinic? Tech Coloproctol. 2017;21:1–4.
22. Parekh PJ, Burleson D, Lubin C, Johonson DA. Colon irrigation: effective, safe, and well-tolerated alternative to traditional therapy in the management of refractory chronic constipation. J Clin Gastroenterol Hepatol. 2018;2:1–5.

23. Parè P, Fedorak RN. Systematic review of stimulant and nonstimulant laxatives for the treatment of functional constipation. Can J Gastroenterol Hepatol. 2014;28:549–57.
24. Miner PB Jr, Camilleri M, Burton D, Achenbach H, Wan H, Dragone J, Mellgard B. Prucalopride induces high-amplitude propagating contractions in the colon of patients with chronic constipation: a randomized study. Neurogastroenterol Motil. 2016;28:1341–8.
25. Krogh K, Bach Jensen M, Gandrup P, Laurberg S, Nilsson J, Kerstens R, De Pauw M. Efficacy and tolerability of prucalopride in patients with constipation due to spinal cord injury. Scand J Gastroenterol. 2002;37:431–6.
26. Roarty TP, Weber F, Soykan I, McCallum RW. Misoprostol in the treatment of chronic refractory constipation: results of a long-term open label trial. Aliment Pharmacol Ther. 1997;11:1059–66.
27. Hawkyard CV, Koerner RJ. The use of erythromycin as a gastrointestinal prokinetic agent in adult critical care: benefits versus risks. J Antimicrob Chemother. 2007;59:347–58.
28. Menarini M, Orlandi S, Geccherle A, Bocus P, Bazzocchi G. Efficacia della procedura di Irrigazione Trans Anale con il dispositivo Qufora-PMC nel trattamento della stipsi severa. Pelviperineologia. 2017;36:3–8.
29. Christensen P, Bazzocchi G, Coggrave M, Abel R, Hultling C, Krogh K, Media S, Laurberg S. Treatment of fecal incontinence and constipation in patients with spinal cord injury: a prospective, randomized, controlled, multicenter trial of transanal irrigation vs conservative bowel management. Gastroenterology. 2006;131:738–47.
30. Midrio P, Mosiello G, Ausili E, Gamba P, Marte A, Lombardi L, Iacobelli BD, Caponcelli E, Marrello S, Meroni M, Brisighelli G, Leva E, Rendeli C. Peristeen transanal irrigation in paediatric patients with anorectal malformations and spinal cord lesions: a multicentre Italian study. Color Dis. 2016;18:86–93.
31. Bazzocchi G, Poletti E, Avogadri A. L'irrigazione retrograda transanale per il bowel management del paziente con lesione midollare mediante dispositive a pressione costante: razionale e procedura per l'utilizzo del Peristeen. Pelviperineology. 2012;31:85–92.
32. Christensen P, Bazzocchi G, Coggrave M, Abel R, Hultling C, Krogh K, Media S, Laurberg S. Outcome of transanal irrigation for bowel dysfunction in patients with spinal cord injury? J Spinal Cord Med. 2008;31:560–7.
33. Emmanuel AV, Krogh K, Bazzocchi G, Leroi AM, Bremers A, Leder D, van Kuppevelt D, Mosiello G, Vogel M, Perrouin-Verbe B, Coggrave M, Christensen P. Consensus review of best practice of transanal irrigation in adults. Spinal Cord. 2013;51:732–8.

Management of the Suprapontine Neurogenic Lower Urinary Tract Dysfunction

8

Gaetano De Rienzo, Gianfranco Lamberti, Luisa De Palma, Donatella Giraudo, Elena Bertolucci, Giuseppina Gibertini, Caterina Gruosso, and Roberta Robol

8.1 Pharmacotherapy

In the case of suprapontine lesions, the most common bladder dysfunction is neurogenic detrusor overactivity. Antimuscarinics can be considered the mainstay of treatment, while other therapies like cannabinoids look promising. Intravesical injection of botulinum toxin can be considered the main second-line treatment in case of failure of antimuscarinics. Conservative treatments should be associated with drugs. Cognitive effects of therapy shall be bared in mind for all the therapies with systemic absorption.

G. De Rienzo
Urology and Andrology Unit II, University of Bari, Bari, Italy

G. Lamberti (✉)
Neurorehabilitation Unit and Pelvic Floor Dysfunction Rehabilitation Center, SS Trinità Hospital, Cuneo, Italy

L. De Palma
UOC MFR and Unipolar Spinal Unit, Polyclinic Consortium Hospital of Bari, Bari, Italy

D. Giraudo
Urology Department, San Raffaele Turro Hospital, Milan, Italy
e-mail: giraudo.donatella@hsr.it

E. Bertolucci · G. Gibertini
Neuro-Urology Unit, CTO - Spinal Unit, Città della Salute e della Scienza di Torino, Turin, Italy
e-mail: ggibertini@cittadellasalute.to.it

C. Gruosso
University of Rome Tor Vergata, Rome, Italy

R. Robol
ASST dei Sette Laghi, Hospital "Del Ponte", Varese, Italy

© Springer Nature Switzerland AG 2020
G. Lamberti et al. (eds.), *Suprapontine Lesions and Neurogenic Pelvic Dysfunctions*, Urodynamics, Neurourology and Pelvic Floor Dysfunctions, https://doi.org/10.1007/978-3-030-29775-6_8

As specified in the chapter dedicated to the pathophysiology of LUTD in suprapontine lesions, the predominant clinical condition consists of UI due to detrusor overactivity (DO), associated to detrusor underactivity (DU) in a minority of patients. Sphincter incompetence is quite infrequent as well, and the clinical phenotype consists of urge incontinence too [1–5].

The pharmacotherapy of incontinence in suprapontine lesions consists of the typical spectrum of drugs commonly used in OAB; their integration with conservative treatment is often the key of successful treatment, as these patients can experience limitations in movements and/or cognitive impairment concurring to the occurrence and maintaining of incontinence [6].

8.2 Antimuscarinics

Micturition in suprapontine lesions is usually coordinated, and then in this category of patients the symptom relief is the primary intent of treatment. In general, the evidence base for their use in the neurogenic bladder is limited, and data about the suprapontine disease are scarce and usually limited to Parkinson's disease (PD) and cerebrovascular accidents (CVA) [7].

Special attention is needed in case of cognition impairment, as antimuscarinics can cause deterioration in memory or onset of confusion.

Oxybutynin hydrochloride has shown adequate efficacy and safety profile in Parkinson's disease and multiple sclerosis, when used with titration criteria, until the dosage of the maximum therapeutic effect/tolerability balance is reached, even at a dosage of 30 mg per day [8].

When compared to oxybutynin, propiverine shows similar urodynamic and symptomatic improvement, but with a lower incidence of dry mouth [9].

Trospium chloride has shown urodynamic and clinical improvement in neurogenic detrusor overactivity (NDO) while not passing the blood-brain barrier (BBB). This is at least in theory an advantage for suprapontine lesions in case of cognitive impairment.

Solifenacin has been extensively studied in neurogenic DO, mostly in MS and spinal cord injuries, showing efficacy in urodynamic parameter improvements (first desire, volume at first involuntary contraction, maximum cystometric capacity), symptom relief and reduction of incontinence. A trial also exists, addressing the reduction of micturitions/24 h in PD pts. with OAB. In this study, the reduction in incontinence episodes is a secondary endpoint, while cognitive effects were not explored [10].

Very few data exist about darifenacin and fesoterodine in NDO.

Association of two different AM (usually a combination of oxybutynin, tolterodine and trospium) has shown to be effective and well tolerated, but data are limited to understand if the safety profile is increased [11].

Only one study has explored the eventuality of reducing the cognitive effects of AM by the use of central acetylcholinesterase inhibitors. The results of the

Mini-Mental State Examination (MMSE) and ADAS-cog led the authors to conclude that this association could be an option in case of association of dementia and OAB [12].

8.3   Mirabegron

Mirabegron is the only representative of a new family of drugs addressing OAB. Mirabegron is a β3 agonist with adequate selectivity (even if not exclusive) for bladder adrenoceptors.

Several reports exist about NDO in case of SI and MS, while data about suprapontine DO are more sparse. We could identify at least one study by Chen who showed symptom improvement in the absence of modifications of PVR and voided volumes, in 66 patients with CVA, PD, and dementia. Only two dropouts were registered due to the absence of therapeutic effects [13, 14].

Mirabegron should not produce cognitive impairment. β3 Receptors are present in the brain, but their function is still unclear.

8.4   Cannabinoid Agonists

Oral cannabinoid agents have shown a relaxing effect on bowel and bladder, tested in open-label as well as randomised clinical trials in SM patients. Specific data about suprapontine diseases are missing; experimental studies suggest that exocannabinoids and endocannabinoids could act at urothelial level, regulating afferent transmission [15–18].

8.5   Botulinum Toxin

Intravesical administration of onabotulinumtoxinA is a well-established second-line therapy when AM fails. In randomised multicentre trial complete continence was achieved in 36–38% of pts. with a 200UI toxin (40–41% with 300UI), while single-centre studies and one real-life study showed higher success rates. The therapy produces a significant quality-of-life improvement [19–21].

Focusing on suprapontine diseases, the most studied pathologies were Parkinson's disease and cerebrovascular accident. In these patients BotoxA showed symptom and urodynamic efficacy. Data about long-term efficacy are rare: in extension study of registration trials, QoL was maintained at 3 years with repeat injections [24–27].

The treatment is overall safe, with urinary retention needing de novo CIC as the most concerning side effect (30–47%) [19, 21]. Haematuria and UTI are minor side effects, while the most serious event of generalised fatigue was observed in 0.005% only of cases, spontaneously resolving in 3–4 weeks [21–23].

8.6 Percutaneous and Transcutaneous Tibial Nerve Stimulation

Different pathologies of the central nervous system can cause neuro-urological symptoms. The neuro-urological symptoms depend on the location of the disease and the extent of the neurological lesion. Correctly, the suprapontine lesions are characterised by the interruption of inhibitory inputs to the CPM (pontine micturition centre); pathologies such as cerebrovascular lesions, Parkinson's disease, tumours and traumatic brain injury and multiple sclerosis (depending on the location and severity of the lesion), determine an uncontrolled detrusor activity that results clinically in a neurogenic overactive bladder with symptoms such as voiding frequency, urgency, urge incontinence and nocturia. For example, in patients with Alzheimer's disease, around 25% is reached, and up to 100% in patients who have advanced sclerosis. Neurogenic dysfunctions of the low urinary tract (NLUTD) substantially compromise the quality of life of the neuro-urological patient.

Percutaneous tibial nerve stimulation (PTNS) is a neuromodulation technique for treating symptoms of the lower urinary tract, obtained by electrical stimulation of the posterior tibial nerve. It is introduced as an alternative treatment for all those patients who are resistant to conservative therapies. The first to study its effects in 1983 was McGuire [24], who observed some improvement in symptoms in patients with lower urinary tract dysfunction (LUTS), stimulating the posterior tibial nerve and the common peroneal nerve, with adhesive electrodes. He demonstrated that transcutaneous electrical stimulation of the posterior tibial nerve could eliminate detrusor overactivity on a neurogenic basis. Subsequently, in the 1990s Stoller [25] and collaborators improved a treatment protocol and described a transdermal stimulation called Stoller afferent stimulation (SANS), a percutaneous stimulation of the posterior tibial nerve for the treatment of overactive bladder (OAB).

The mechanism of action is still unclear [26], but it is assumed that PTNS modulates the signals arriving and departing from the bladder (S2–S3) with afferent and efferent stimulation, through the sacral plexus; not only there are probably central-type paths for which stimulation is afferent retrograde, but there would also be a plastic reorganisation of the cortical network triggered by peripheral neuromodulation [27].

The posterior tibial nerve is in close association with the posterior tibial artery and is a mixed nerve containing motor and sensory fibres, which originates from the L4–S3 nerve roots; these same roots innervate the detrusor, the urinary sphincter and all the pelvic floor muscles.

The patient is placed in the supine position for the stimulation procedure with the knees abducted and bent and the hips in external rotation (frog position); the introduction of a 34-gauge needle is planned approximately 4–5 cm cranially to the medial malleolus, between the posterior margin of the tibia and the soleus muscle [28]. A self-adhesive ground electrode is applied ipsilaterally near the medial calcaneus (Fig. 8.1).

The transcutaneous method (TTNS, performed with two self-adhesive electrodes) (Fig. 8.2) has the advantage that it can be easily performed at home, by the

Fig. 8.1 Percutaneous tibial nerve stimulation (PTNS)

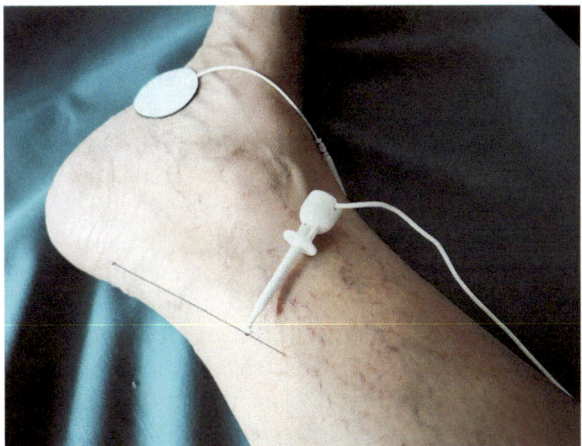

Fig. 8.2 Transcutaneous tibial nerve stimulation (TTNS)

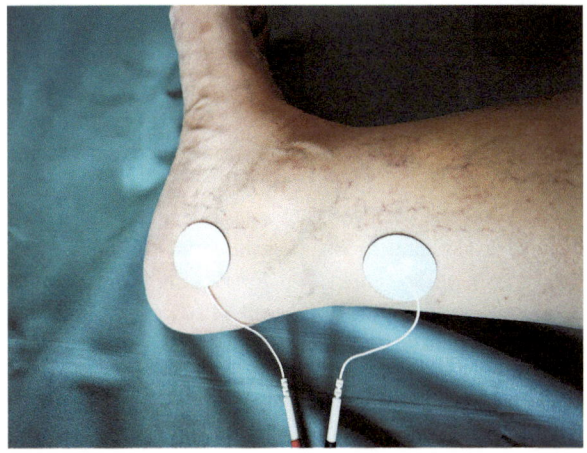

patient or by the caregiver, compared to the percutaneous method, which requires the insertion of the needle near the tibial nerve by a healthcare professional. The effectiveness of the two different stimulation approaches was compared by Ramirez Garcia et al. which demonstrated the non-inferiority of TTNS technique in decreasing the voiding frequency in patients with detrusor overactivity [29].

The point where the needle is introduced was already known by traditional Chinese medicine [30], the SP6 point, as the point for bladder regulation and to relieve pelvic symptoms. A recent study by Yang et al. [31] however would have shown how the stimulation of the BL33 point (very close to S3) is equally effective in inhibiting the overactive bladder.

After positioning the needle, an electrode is placed on the ipsilateral heel bone. The needle and the electrode are both connected to a low-voltage stimulator of about 9 V. The generator that delivers the electrical impulse has fixed stimulation parameters: 200 µs pulse range, 20 Hz pulse frequency and variable stimulus intensity between 0.5 and 9 mA, respecting the patient's tolerance threshold. To confirm the correct positioning of the needle, the power of the stimulus is slowly increased until the bending of the big toe and/or the waving of the other fingers is obtained. Furthermore, patients report a sensitive response to stimulation, such as tingling in the soles of the feet or fingers [32]. The commonly used protocol involves a session per week lasting about 30 min for 10–12 weeks; in this regard, there are studies in the literature that show the same effectiveness, in less time, for more frequent applications [33, 34]. The results seem to depend on the number of stimulations performed but not on time elapsed since the start of the stimulation programme.

The more significant advantage of this technique is that it is minimally invasive; it is not a surgical technique and does not require a permanent stimulation implant as in sacral neuromodulation. The efficacy and safety of sacral neuromodulation techniques (SNM) and percutaneous tibial nerve stimulation (PTNS) were assessed in a recent review [35]: the SNM proves more active, with an improvement rate of symptoms of LUTDs between 61% and 90% while the PTNS rate has a range of around 59–74%. SMN also shows long-term efficacy compared to PTNS, on which unfortunately there are no studies, in this review, on long-term follow-ups, although a 2018 study by Vecchioli-Scaldazza et al. [36] would show that the association of TPNS and solifenacin may have better and more long-term effects than with PTNS therapy alone. The substantial difference between the methods therefore lies in the safety parameters: in NMS there are no significant complications but the most common adverse event, estimated at 15% up to 42%, is pain in the implant; other complications related to surgery and implantation of the stimulator are related to the migration of the same (with consequent reoperation) or the rupture of the cables or a possible infection. Studies on TPNS instead do not report any adverse event and no complication; the only events reported in the studies report minor bleeding and a temporary feeling of pain in the needle application area. There are no surgical procedures required to solve these complications.

In recent years we have witnessed an evolution of the devices for sacral neuromodulation and an attempt has been made to solve the safety issue by implanting increasingly miniaturised electrodes, thus opting for a minimally invasive surgical treatment. The electrode, in this case, is connected to a wireless Bluetooth system [37], which allows it to be recharged and used by an external device. In 2018, AUA proposed a system to the ICS assembly that does not even foresee an external generator. MacDiarmid and collaborators [38] presented a preliminary report of a 12-week prospective, multicentre study on a new implantable system; the device is in titanium, is battery powered and of the size of a coin that can be programmed for home treatment of PTNS. Despite the research efforts, any implant, even the most miniaturised one, is not yet compatible with NMR. PTNS instead, not envisaging any permanent implant, is the only therapy, to date, that does not set these limits. The need to use an NMR-compatible technique is fundamental in the treatment of neurological patients with lower urinary tract dysfunctions on which urinary symptoms have a severe impact on the quality of life. In neurological patients it is the localisation and nature [39] of the neurological lesion that determine the level of dysfunction. The prevalence of neurogenic dysfunction of the lower urinary tract (NLUTD) depends on the neurological disorder; for example in patients with Alzheimer's disease approximately 25% is reached and up to 100% in patients who have advanced multiple sclerosis. NLUTDs represent a significant impairment [40] in the daily life of the neuro-urological patient, substantially compromising the quality of life of the patient.

The use of electrical stimulation in NLUDT is based on a study by Sundin et al. [41] of 1974 in which it is shown that electrical stimulation of the pudendal nerve causes an inhibitory response on the bladder detrusor, in cats. This technique later evolved considerably and was improved and extended to different stimulation areas and is still used as transcutaneous electrical nerve stimulation for the treatment of various neuro-urological dysfunctions. A systematic review of the literature by Gross et al. [42] shows that electrical stimulation determines a positive and safe effect even in neurological patients with LUDT. Concerning PTNS, the number of reports is scarce, especially for patients with a neurological bladder. A trial by Amarenco and colleagues [43] shows an acute effect of PTNS on urodynamics in neuro-injured patients, all with symptoms of overactive bladder syndrome (multiple sclerosis, Parkinson's disease and spinal cord injury); during electrical stimulation there is a significant increase in volume at the first involuntary detrusor contraction and an increase in cystometric capacity. As already pointed out previously, the urinary tract dysfunction is determined by the area and nature of the lesion: for example, the suprapontine lesions [25] will see a predominance of symptoms linked to bladder filling with detrusor overactivity. A publication by Phé et al. [44] on the treatment of PTNS on patients with multiple sclerosis illustrates the effectiveness of treatment in filling symptoms and urodynamic improvement. It reports data from a multicentre study on 70 patients with MS and overactive bladder symptoms. All patients received tibial nerve stimulation for 20 min a day for 3 months. Clinical improvement of symptoms was assessed based on criteria of improvement of frequency/urgency symptoms, patient-self-reported symptoms, bladder control and increased quality of life; in 2017 Canbaz Kabay et al. [45] went the extra mile in treating patients affected by multiple sclerosis with detrusor overactivity (DO) for up to 12 months. He shows that the results obtained with a 3-month treatment are preserved for up to 12 months in patients enrolled in his study. Patients are treated at intervals of 14 days for 3 months, then at an interval of 21 days for the following 3 months, and finally at an interval of 28 days. The protocol used by Kabay involves the introduction of a 26-gauge needle inserted about 5 cm cranially to the medial malleolus and an electrode on the ipsilateral heel bone. The stimulation is applied unilaterally using 200 µs pulse range, 20 Hz pulse frequency and variable stimulus intensity between 1 and 5 mA, observing the tolerance threshold of the patient and in any case capable of evoking foot bending or waving of the fingers. All parametric variables of daily micturition, frequency, urgency and nocturia and episodes of incontinence appear significantly improved compared to the baseline, as well as the perception of the quality of life.

Some symptoms of the lower urinary tract such as urgency, daytime frequency and nocturia are also very common in autonomic disorder in patients with Parkinson's disease (PD). Urodynamic alterations and functional abnormalities, including neurogenic overactivity of the detrusor (hyporeflexia or areflexia), affect the performance of the external sphincter. In this sense, a study by Kabay [46] highlights how a 12-week treatment with percutaneous stimulation of the posterior tibial nerve, PTNS, produced a statistically significant improvement in LUTS and urodynamic parameters in PD patients. The parameters used in the study included urodynamic measurements before and after 12 weeks of treatment with PTNS; short questionnaire form (ICIQ-SF); and overactive bladder questionnaire (OAB-V8). The protocol used is the same, parameterised to fixed stimulation stimuli as described in the literature.

Contrary to motor disorders, many PD patients are not responders to levodopa treatment for LUTS, which is why non-invasive treatment with PTNS could be a proposal to all those PD patients whose other conservative therapies have failed to respond significantly.

As we know, the exact mechanism and effect of PTNS on the neurological bladder are not yet clear; the study by Finazzi-Agrò [47] reports the effect on the supraspinal centres reporting a significant increase in the magnitude of somatosensory evoked potentials to long latency recorded 24 h after the end of a PTNS programme session. This discovery could reflect a change in the processing mechanisms of sensory stimuli and suggests a possible reorganisation of cortical excitability after PTNS. Improvement, especially concerning the overactive bladder, is an encouraging result that suggests the stimulation of the posterior tibial nerve as a non-invasive treatment method in patients with the neurological bladder.

8.7 Bladder Catheterism

The suprapontine neurological bladder is the consequence of lesions in both cerebral hemispheres, particularly in the frontal lobes (multi-infarct encephalopathy, brain atrophy, tumours, brain traumas, hydrocephalus) or in the basal ganglia (Parkinson's disease and multiple system atrophy).

Brain suffering causes a reduction in inhibitory control that is exercised under physiological conditions on the urination pontine centre; consequently an uncontrolled detrusor activity is established, defined as "neurogenic detrusor overactivity". Patients are affected by non-inhibited detrusor contractions that cause an increase in voiding frequency, reduction in the ability to delay the voiding action after the appearance of the first stimulus (urgency) and an "urgency" incontinence. The post-voiding bladder residue, i.e. the amount of urine that remains in the bladder after urination, is absent or insignificant (less than 80 mL); diseases that most frequently involve this condition are cerebral thrombosis and haemorrhages, dementia (Alzheimer's, Pick), brain tumours and hydrocephalus.

Urinary disorders in patients with Parkinson's disease generally appear in late stages of the disease and are related to the depletion of dopaminergic neurons in the black substance and the subsequent reduction of striatal dopamine. Thus, secondary detrusor overactivity and reduced D1 mediated tonic inhibitory activity are determined. An alternative hypothesis is the presence of a neurotransmitter imbalance of neurons, with a facilitating action on the urination pontine centre, the ventral tegmental area that would cause pollakiuria (urination for low volumes of bladder filling), nocturia (repeated nocturnal urination) and urination urgency. In addition to detrusor overactivity, in Parkinson's disease, there is also a delayed relaxation of the perineal musculature at the beginning of the voiding action (bradykinesia of the striatum external urethral sphincter) and a detrusor muscle contractility deficit, secondary to anti-Parkinsonian drug therapy, which can cause partial urinary retention.

8.8 Frequency of Catheterisation

In the assessment of the patient trained in catheterisation (Table 8.1), the volume of spontaneous urination and the residual volume must be monitored by recording them in a diary; in this way, the frequency of execution of the IC can be determined.

As a general rule, residual volumes of urine in adults must not exceed 500 mL. However, the guidelines on the subject can also be based on bladder capacity, detrusor pressure in the filling phase, presence of reflux and renal function [48].

If the patient is unable to urinate independently, it is usually necessary to repeat the IC from 4 to 6 times a day to obtain a bladder volume between 300 and 500 mL.

Excessive fluid intake increases the risk of bladder overdilation and incontinence due to regurgitation.

Table 8.1 Initial management of neurogenic urinary incontinence

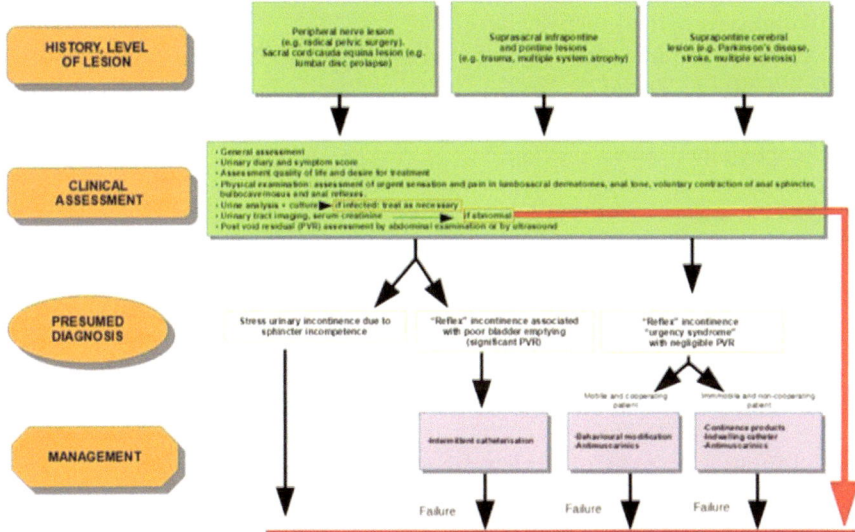

8.9   Recommendations

- Evaluate the patient's fluid intake in the presence of urine production of >3 L/day or if it is necessary to use catheterisation> six times/day >>. Level 4, grade C.
- Evaluate the fluid intake by the patient in the presence of urine production of >500 mL per catheterisation. Level 4, grade C.
- Evaluate the frequency of IC in the presence of urine production of >500 mL per catheterisation. Level 4, grade C.
- Evaluate the need to adapt treatment with antimuscarinic drugs in patients with residual post-urination urine volumes (PVR) and bladder hyperactivity (OAB), as well as the need for frequent catheterisation. Level 4, grade C.
- IC is recommended before going to bed to help reduce nocturia. Level 4, grade C.
- Ultrasound is used in measuring the residual volume of urine following spontaneous emptying of the bladder. Level 4, grade C.

8.10   Patients and Caregivers

Patients and caregivers must be evaluated concerning:

- General health conditions
- Knowledge of the urinary tract
- Ability to understand information
- Ability to use their knowledge
- Compliance
- The need for psychological support
- Motivation and emotional readiness
- Willingness to implement the procedure
- Adapting the frequency of catheterisation; if the catheterisation volume is <100 mL or >500 mL
- Adapting the catheterisation intervals
- Adapting fluid intake

References

1. Powell CR. Not all neurogenic bladders are the same: a proposal for a new neurogenic bladder classification system. Transl Androl Urol. 2016;5:12–21.
2. Griffiths D. In: Vodusek DB, editor. Functional imaging of structures involved in the neural control of the LUT. Amsterdam: Elsevier; 2015.
3. De Groat WC, Griffiths D, Yoshimura N. Neural control of the lower urinary tract. Compr Physiol. 2015;5:327–96.
4. Sakakibara R. In: Vodusek DB, editor. Lower urinary tract dysfunction in patients with brain lesions. 1st ed. Amsterdam: Elsevier; 2015.
5. Mehnert U. Neuro-urological dysfunction of the lower urinary tract in CNS diseases: pathophysiology, epidemiology and treatment options. Urologe. 2012;51:189–97.

6. Panicker JN. Lower urinary tract symptoms following neurological illness may be influenced by multiple factors: observations from a neurorehabilitation service in a developing country. Neurourol Urodyn. 2010;29:378–81.
7. Nicholas RS. Anticholinergics for urinary symptoms in multiple sclerosis. Cochrane Database Syst Rev. 2009:CD004193.
8. Bennett N. Can higher doses of oxybutynin improve efficacy in the neurogenic bladder? J Urol. 2004;171:749–51.
9. Stohrer M. Propiverine compared to oxybutynin in neurogenic detrusor overactivity: results of a randomised, double-blind, multicenter clinical study. Eur Urol. 2007;51:235–42.
10. Zasiewics TA. Randomized, controlled pilot trial of solifenacin succinate for overactive bladder in Parkinson's disease. Parkinsonism Relat Disord. 2015;21:14–20.
11. Amend B. Effective treatment of neurogenic detrusor dysfunction by combined high dosed antimuscarinics without increased side effects. Eur Urol. 2008;53:1021–8.
12. Sakakibara R. How to manage overactive bladder in elderly individuals with dementia? A combined use of donepezil, a central acetylcholinesterase inhibitor, and propiverine, a peripheral muscarine receptor antagonist. J Am Geriatr Soc. 2009;57:1515–7.
13. Wollner J. Initial experience with the treatment of neurogenic detrusor overactivity with a new beta-3 agonist (Mirabegron) in patients with spinal cord injury. Spinal Cord. 2016;54: 78–82.
14. Chen SF. Therapeutic efficacy of low-dose (25 mg) mirabegron therapy for patients with mild to moderate overactive bladder symptoms due to central nervous system diseases. Low Urin Tract Symptoms. 2018;5:1–6.
15. Brady CM. An open-label study of cannabis-based extracts for bladder dysfunction in advanced multiple sclerosis. Mult Scler. 2004;10:425–33.
16. Freeman RM. The effect of cannabis on urge incontinence in patients with multiple sclerosis: a multicenter, randomised placebo-controlled trial (CAMS-LUTS). Int Urogynecol J Pelvic Floor Dysfunct. 2006;17:636–41.
17. Strittmatter F. Expression of fatty acid amide hydrolase (FAAH) in human, mouse, and rat urinary bladder and effects of FAAH inhibition on bladder function in awake rats. Eur Urol. 2012;61:98–106.
18. Aizawa N. Inhibition of peripheral FAAH depresses activities of bladder mechanosensitive nerve fibers of the rat. J Urol. 2014;192:956–63.
19. Cruz F. Efficacy and safety of continence due to neurogenic detrusor overactivity: a randomised, double-blind, placebo-controlled trial. Eur Urol. 2011;60:472–50.
20. Herschorn S. Efficacy of botulinum toxin A injection for neurogenic detrusor overactivity and urinary incontinence: a randomised, double blind trial. J Urol. 2011;185:2229–35.
21. Ginsberg D. Phase 3 efficacy and tolerability study of onabotulinumtoxinA for urinary incontinence from neurogenic detrusor overactivity. J Urol. 2012;187:2131–9.
22. Del Popolo G. Neurogenic detrusor overactivity treated with English botulinum toxin A: 8-year experience of one single centre. Eur Urol. 2008;53:1013–20.
23. De Laet K. Adverse events after botulinum A toxin injection for neurogenic voiding disorders. Spinal Cord. 2005;43:397–9.
24. Groen J, Pannek J, Castro Diaz D, et al. Summary of European association of urology (EAU) guidelines on neuro-urology. Eur Urol. 2016;69:324–33.
25. Panicker JN, Fowler CJ, Kessler TM. Lower urinary tract dysfunction in the neurological patient: clinical assessment and management. Lancet Neurol. 2015;14:720–32.
26. McGuire E, Zhang S, Horwinski E, Lytton B. Treatment of motor and sensory detrusor instability by electrical stimulation. J Urol. 1983;129(1):78–9.
27. Finazzi-Agrò E, Rocchi C, Pachats C, et al. Percutaneous tibial nerve stimulation produces effects on brain activity: study on the modifications of the long latency somatosensory evoked potentials. Neurourol Urodyn. 2009;28(4):320–4.
28. Stoller M. Afferent nerve stimulation for pelvic floor dysfunction. Eur Urol. 1999;35 (Suppl 2):16.

29. Ramírez-García I, Blanco-Ratto L, Kauffmann S, et al. Efficacy of transcutaneous stimulation of the posterior tibial nerve compared to percutaneous stimulation in idiopathic overactive bladder syndrome: randomised control trial. Neurourol Urodyn. 2018;37:1–8.

30. Chang P. Urodynamic studies in acupuncture for women with frequency, urgency and dysuria. J Urol. 1988;140(3):563–6.

31. Yang L, Wang Y, Mo Q. A comparative study of electroacupunture at Zhongliao (BL33) and other acupoint for overactive bladder symptoms. Front Med. 2017;11(1):129–36.

32. MacDiarmid SA, Staskin DR. Percutaneous tibial nerve stimulation (PTNS): a literature-based assessment. Curr Bladder Dysfunct Rep. 2009;4(1):29–33.

33. Matthew R, Cooperberg T, Stoller ML. Percutaneous neuromodulation. Urol Clin N Am. 2005;32:71–8.

34. Finazzi A, Campagna A, Sciobica F, et al. Posterior tibial nerve stimulation: is the once-a-week protocol the best option? Minerva Nefrol. 2005;57:119–23.

35. Martin-Garcia M, Crampton J. A single-blind, randomised controlled trial to evaluate the effectiveness of transcutaneous tibial nerve stimulation (TTNS) in overactive bladder symptoms in women responders to percutaneous tibial nerve stimulation (PTNS). Physiotherapy. 2018; https://doi.org/10.1016/j.physio.2018.12.002.

36. Vecchioli-Scaldazza C. Effectiveness and durability of solifenacin versus percutaneous tibial nerve stimulation versus their combination for the treatment of women with overactive bladder syndrome: a randomised controlled study with a follow-up of ten months. Int Braz J Urol. 2018;44:102–8.

37. Heesakkers J, Digesu G, van Breda J, et al. A novel leadless, miniature implantable Tibial nerve neuromodulation system for the management of overactive bladder complaints. Neurourol Urodyn. 2018;37:1060–7.

38. MacDiarmid S, Lucente V, Kaaki B, et al. Safety & efficacy of the eCoin™ implantable tibial nerve stimulation device for overactive bladder syndrome: UroToday. p. MP75–18.

39. Van Balken M, Vergunst H, Bemelmans B. The use of electrical devices for the treatment of bladder dysfunction: a review of methods. J Urol. 2004;172:846–51.

40. Yoong W, Ridout AE, Damodaram M, et al. Neuromodulative treatment with percutaneous tibial nerve stimulation for intractable detrusor instability: outcomes following a shortened 6-week protocol. BJU Int. 2010;106:1673–6.

41. Sundin T, Carlsson CA, Kock NG. Detrusor inhibition induced from mechanical stimulation of the anal region and from electrical stimulation of pudendal nerve afferents. An experimental study in cats. Investig Urol. 1974;11:374–8.

42. Gross T, Schneider M, Bachmann L, et al. Transcutaneous electrical nerve stimulation for treating neurogenic lower urinary tract dysfunction: a systematic review. Eur Urol. 2016;69:1102–11.

43. Amarenco G, Ismael SS, Even-Schneider A, et al. Urodynamic effect of acute transcutaneous posterior tibial nerve stimulation in overactive bladder. J Urol. 2003;169:2210–5.

44. Phé V, Chartier-Kastler E, Panicker JN. Management of neurogenic bladder in patients with multiple sclerosis. Nat. Rev Urol. 2016 May;13(5):275–88. https://doi.org/10.1038/nrurol.2016.53.

45. Canbaz Kabay S, Kabay S, Mestan E, Cetiner M, Ayas S, Sevim M, Ozden H, Karaman HO. Long term sustained therapeutic effects of percutaneous posterior tibial nerve stimulation treatment of neurogenic overactive bladder in multiple sclerosis patients: 12-months results. Neurourol Urodyn. 2017;36(1):104–10.

46. Kabay S, Canbaz Kabay S, Cetiner M, et al. The Clinical and Urodynamic Results of Percutaneous Posterior Tibial Nerve Stimulation on Neurogenic Detrusor Overactivity in Patients With Parkinson's Disease. Urology. 2016;87:76–81.

47. Finazzi-Agrò E, Rocchi C, Pachats C, et al. Percutaneous Tibial nerve stimulation produces effects on brain activity: study on the modifications of the long latency somatosensory evoked potentials. Neurourol Urodyn. 2009;28(4):320–4.

48. Vahr S, Cobussen-Boekhorst H, Eikenboom J, Geng V, et al. Evidence-based guidelines for best practice in urological health care. Catheterisation urethral intermittent catheterisation in adults. Revised by Biroli A, Gibertini G. Fondazione Italiana Continenza, 2018.

Pelvic Floor Muscle Training and Neurogenic Overactive Bladder in Stroke and Multiple Sclerosis

9

Kari Bø

9.1 Introduction

Pelvic floor muscle training (PFMT) has Level 1 evidence and A recommendation for treatment of urinary incontinence (UI) in the female population [1–3]. The Cochrane review [1] on 31 randomized controlled trials (RCTs)/quasi RCTs in 1817 women from 14 countries compared PFMT with no treated control groups in trials of women with stress urinary incontinence (SUI), urgency urinary incontinence (UUI), and mixed urinary incontinence (MUI). Women with SUI who did PFMT were eight times more likely to report cure (56% vs. 6%; risk ratio (RR) 8.38, 95% confidence interval (CI) 3.68–19.07). They had statistically significant better improvement in quality of life (QoL), fewer UI episodes, and less UI on pad test compared to controls. The effect was higher in women with SUI only and with supervised training. Based on this evidence and that PFMT has no adverse effects, PFMT is recommended as first-line treatment for UI in women [1–3]. RCTs of PFMT on UI in men have so far focused on post-prostatectomy incontinence [1, 2]. However, the results differ and are not as convincing as for women, although single RCTs with high methodological and interventional quality have found statistically significant and clinically relevant results [4].

The rationale for PFMT to treat and prevent SUI is that strength training of the muscles will improve structural support of the bladder and urethra by lifting the pelvic floor higher into the pelvis, narrow the levator hiatus area, prevent descent during rise in intra-abdominal pressure, and increase maximum urethral closure pressure [5]. Such morphological changes have been shown in an assessor-blinded RCT [6]. The rationale for PFMT to prevent and treat OAB

K. Bø (✉)

Department of Sports Medicine, Norwegian School of Sport Sciences, Oslo, Norway

Department of Obstetrics and Gynecology, Akershus University Hospital, Akershus, Norway

e-mail: kari.bo@nih.no

© Springer Nature Switzerland AG 2020

G. Lamberti et al. (eds.), *Suprapontine Lesions and Neurogenic Pelvic Dysfunctions*, Urodynamics, Neurourology and Pelvic Floor Dysfunctions, https://doi.org/10.1007/978-3-030-29775-6_9

symptoms is based on a theory that contraction of the PFM will inhibit urgency to void and detrusor contraction [7]. Shafic and Shafic [8] found a significant decrease in detrusor pressure and increase in urethral pressure and no leakage in patients with OAB symptoms during a single PFM contraction during urgency. However, to date there is no strong evidence from RCTs that PFMT alone is effective in treatment of overactive bladder (OAB) symptoms (nocturia, frequency, urgency, and (UUI) [7].

UI is prevalent in the general population and causes distress and reduced quality of life [9]. In patients with neurological diseases this adds to the total burden of an illness with reduced mobility. UI may be caused by neurological diseases and be the first symptom of such conditions, but many of these patients may also have different forms of UI caused by other factors before they present with neurological diseases such as stroke, multiple sclerosis (MS), or Parkinson's disease.

The aim of this chapter is to review the scientific literature of RCTs on PFMT after stroke and in patients with MS and Parkinson's disease. Furthermore it aims to give some recommendations to guide clinical practice and future clinical research.

9.2 Methods

This is a narrative review on PFMT for UI in patients after stroke and patients with MS and Parkinson's disease. Search on Cochrane library of systematic reviews, NICE guidelines, and the chapter of Van Kampen and Geraerts in Evidence based physical therapy for teh pelvic floor. Bridging science and clinical prcatice [10]— were used to find relevant studies of PFMT for UI in patients with stroke, MS, and Parkinson's disease. In addition, search for new studies on PubMed of May 2019 using the terms stroke AND pelvic floor muscle training or multiple sclerosis or AND pelvic floor muscle training was performed. Only randomized controlled trials written in English language were included. The interventions could include PFMT alone or a combination of other conservative interventions such as bladder training, electrical stimulation, or transcutaneous tibial nerve stimulation. Studies including pharmacotherapy were excluded.

9.3 Results

No randomized controlled trials were found of PFMT on UI in patients with Parkinson's disease. This was supported by a recent systematic review on management of neurogenic bladder in Parkinson's disease that only found two pilot studies, one on PFMT and one on bladder training. Their conclusion was that well-designed RCTs are needed [11]. One Cochrane review from 2008 was found on treatment of UI after stroke [12]. Results of the RCTs of PFMT for UI in patients with stroke or MS are shown in Tables 9.1 and 9.2.

Table 9.1 Randomized controlled trials (RCTs) of pelvic floor muscle training (PFMT) for urinary incontinence (UI) in stroke patients. Chronological order

	Design	Population/N	Diagnosis of UI	Training protocol	Dropout	Adherence	Results on PFM function	Results on UI
Tibaek-04, 05 [13, 14]	Assessor-blinded two-arm RCT: 1. PFMT $n = 14$ 2. Control $n = 12$ No treatment for UI, standard rehabilitation program	26 women. Mean age 60 years (range 56–74) after ischemic stroke	UI assessed by IIQ-7 (urgency, stress, and mixed incontinence)	12 weeks of PFMT 6-, 3-, and 30-s contractions. Every contraction 4–8 times in different positions. Conducted in groups + individual assessment with vaginal palpation and home exercise 1–2 times/day	2 dropouts (8%)		Statistically significant increase in PFM endurance compared with control	Statistically significant improvement in PFMT in frequency of daytime voiding from 7 to 6 ($p = 0.018$), 24-h pad test from 8 to 2 g ($p = 0.013$) No effect in SF-36 or IIQ-7
Tibaek-07 [15]	6-month follow-up of assessor-blinded RCT 1. PFMT $n = 12$ 2. Control $n = 12$	24 women with postischemic stroke	UI assessed by IIQ-7	Same as Tibaek (2005)	8%			Telephone interview: Trend, but not statistically significant difference between groups in Short form SF-36 or IIQ-7

(continued)

Table 9.1 (continued)

	Design	Population/N	Diagnosis of UI	Training protocol	Dropout	Adherence	Results on PFM function	Results on UI
Shin-16 [16]	Assessor-blinded two-arm RCT: 1. PFMT ($n = 16$) general rehabilitation + PFMT 2. Control ($n = 15$) general rehabilitation	31 female patients >3 months post-stroke	SUI assessed by B-FLUTS	6 weeks of PFMT	3 dropouts		After intervention: Manometry (mmHg): 1. 18.35 (5.24) 2. 8.46 (3.50) sEMG ((μV): 1. 12.09 (2.24) 2. 9.33 (3.40)	B-FLUTS Change of scores: inconvenience: 1. −15.00 (6.25) 2. −0.17 (1.59) Score of symptoms: 1. −4.17 (4.00) 2. −0.25 (1.29) $p < 0.05$
Tibaek-16 Tibaek-17 [17, 18]	Assessor-blinded two-arm RCT 1. Control: General rehabilitation, $n = 15$ 2. General rehabilitation + PFMT, $n = 15$	31 post-stroke men, median age 68		3 months of 12-weekly 60-min sessions of group PFMT with physical therapist including anal assessment + home exercise	1 dropout	Median PFMT adherence 11/12 (92%)	Anal palpation Statistically significant better improvement ($p > 0.03$) in PFM function in PFMT than control in short term, but not long term	DAN-PSS-1: No sign difference in change between groups SF-36 and nocturia QoL questionnaire: No statistically significant difference between groups

B-FUTS Bristol Female Lower Urinary Tract Symptom Questionnaire, *DAN-PSS-1* Danish Prostate Symptom Score, *IIQ-7* Incontinence Impact Questionnaire, *PFM* pelvic floor muscles, *PFMT* pelvic floor muscle training, *QoL* quality of life

Table 9.2 Randomized controlled trials (RCTs) of pelvic floor muscle training (PFMT) on urinary incontinence (UI) in patients with multiple sclerosis (MS. Chronological order)

	Design	N	Diagnosis of UI	Training protocol	Dropout	Adherence	Results PFM function	Results outcome
Vahtera-97 [19]	Not blinded two-arm RCT: 1. PFMT + interferential ES, n = 40 2. No treatment for LUTD, n = 40	50 women and 80 men with MS, age range 25–68	LUTS by self-administered questionnaire	6 months of 10 times 3-s contractions, 5 times 5-s contractions, 5 times 15-s contraction in different positions. ES: interferential, carrier frequency: 2000 Hz, frequency, 5–19 Hz, 10–50 Hz, and 50 Hz (10 min of each). Six sessions during 21 days outpatient. Home exercise: 20 contractions 3–5 days/week in sitting and standing position	2/40 in treatment group No information about controls	62.5%	sEMG Sign improvement over control, p < 0.01	Significant improvement in intervention over control group in UI, nocturia, and urgency p < 0.001, QoL (traveling, social shame, and need for pads)
McClurg-06 [20]	Not blinded three-arm RCT: 1. PFMT + advice n = 10 2. PFMT + advice + EMG biofeedback n = 10 3. PFMT + advice + sEMG biofeedback + ES n = 10	30 women with MS, age range 33–67	Leakage on voiding diary, 24-h pad test, uroflowmetry	9-week treatment period, assessment at weeks 0, 9, 16, 24 ES: biphasic constant current, 5–30 min daily, two parameter settings: 40 Hz, 5-s on, 10-s off 10 Hz, 10-s on, 3-s off	2/30		Vaginal palpation	Number of leaks (p = 0.014) and pad test (p = 0.001) significantly better in group 3 compared to group 1 and between groups 2 and 1 for pad test (p = 0.001)

(continued)

Table 9.2 (continued)

	Design	N	Diagnosis of UI	Training protocol	Dropout	Adherence	Results PFM function	Results outcome
McClurg-08 [21]	Assessor and subject-blinded two-arm RCT: 1. Control: PFMT, biofeedback + placebo ES, n = 37 2. ES: PFMT, biofeedback + ES, n = 37	74 women with MS, age range 27–72	Leakage on voiding diary, 24-h pad test, uroflowmetry	9-week treatment, assessment at weeks 0, 9, 16, 24 ES: biphasic constant current, 5–30 min daily, two parameter settings: 40 Hz, 5-s on, 10-s off 10 Hz, 10-s on, 3-s off	2/74		Vaginal palpation, sEMG	Sign difference in favor of ES for leakage, 24-h pad test
Khan-10 [22]	Not blinded two-arm RCT: 1. Bladder rehab, n = 40 2. Control: usual care, n = 34	74 women with MS, age range 29–65		Inpatient program: 3 h/day over 6 weeks Outpatient program: 30 min 2–3 times/week Therapy: individual, assessment of bladder type, diary with strict fluid, PFMT, timed voiding	22%			Significant difference in favor of intervention in UDI-16, NSD, AUA, IIQ-7 (p < 0.01). Improvement in bladder function, overactivity and QoL

| Lucio-10, -11 [23, 24] | Assessor-blinded two-arm RCT 1. PFMT with vaginal manometry, $n = 18$ 2. Sham PFMT: Insertion of vaginal instrument with no contraction, $n = 17$ | 35 women with MS, age range 20–49 | Lower urinary tract dysfunction assessed with urodynamics | 30 min 2 times/week for 12 weeks (outpatient) PFMT with vaginal manometer: 30 slow contractions, 3 min of fast contractions, supine position. Home exercise: 3×30 slow contractions, 3 min with fast contractions | 22.8% | Vaginal manometry. Statistically significant improvement in muscle strength, endurance, resistance, number of fast contractions, $p < 0.001$ | Between-group differences in favor of PFMT: Pad test: 87.5–6.03 vs. 69.46–75.88, $p < 0.001$ Number of pads: 3.61–2.15 vs. 3.42–3.28, $p = <0.01$ Nocturia events: 2.38–0.46 vs. 2.55–2.47, $p > 0.001$, ICIQ, OAB questionnaire, medical outcome study, QoL: Qualiveen questionnaire. No sign difference in urodynamics |

(continued)

Table 9.2 (continued)

	Design	N	Diagnosis of UI	Training protocol	Dropout	Adherence	Results PFM function	Results outcome
Gaspard-14 [25]	Assessor-blinded RCT: 1. PFMT + biofeedback n = 16 2. Transcutaneous posterior tibia nerve stimulation n = 15	31 participants	EDSS score <7 and lower urinary tract symptoms	9 session of 30 weekly sessions 1. Muscle endurance and relaxation 2. Rectangular alternative biphasic current with low frequency			No information. Article in French. Abstract in English.	Statistically significant improvement in QoL, frequency of urgency episodes, but no difference between groups
Ferreira-15 [26]	Assessor-blinded RCT: 1. PFMT + ES 2. Home PFMT	24 women, mean age 43.2 years (10.68)	Moderate stage of MS, 3.0–5.0 EDSS	48 sessions 2 times / week over 6 months with physical therapist Electrostimulation, 2 Hz, 1 ms pulse duration, tolerable intensity on S4 dermatome- perineum + 3 sets of 10 PFM contractions per day Control group; 10 sets of home PFM contractions per day			Vaginal palpation. Group 1 had statistically significant improvement over the control group in al sub-scores, $p < 0.001$	QoL: Only statistical significant difference in "Restrictions," $p = 0.0031$, OAB: statistically significant difference in change in favor of Group 1, $p = 0.039$. Hospital anxiety and depression: no statistically significant difference between groups

Lucio-16 [27]	Assessor-blinded RCT 1. PFMT with sEMG biofeedback + sham ES, n = 10. 2. PFMT with sEMG biofeedback + ES, n = 10. 3. PFMT with sEMG + transcutaneous tibial nerve stimulation, n = 10	30 women with MS, 42–52 years old	MS with EDSS score <6.5 LUTS: score ≥ 9 on OAB –V8 Urodynamic assessment ICIQ-UI-SF	12-week intervention with physical therapist 50 min twice a week	5 dropouts	Ability to contract PFM: vaginal palpation. Statistically significant improvement in Group 2 in PFM tone, flexibility, ability to relax PFM	24-h pad test: no difference between groups OAB-V8: Group 2 significant improvement over other groups, $p < 0.01$

AUA American Urology Association, *EDSS* Expanded Disability Status Scale in Multiple Sclerosis, *ES* electrical stimulation intravaginal), *ICIQ-UI-SF* International Consultation of Incontinence Questionnaire-urinary incontinence-short form, *LUTS* lower urinary tract symptoms, *NMES* neuromuscular electrical stimulation, *NSD* Neurological Disability Scale, *OAB-V8* Overactive Bladder Questionnaire, version 8, *PFM* pelvic floor muscle, *QoL* quality of life, *sEMG* surface electromyography, *UDI-16* Urogenital Distress Inventory

9.3.1 Stroke

Four RCTs were found on PFMT and stroke from 2004 till 2017 (Table 9.1). The studies came out from two research groups [13–18], and Tibaek et al. conducted three of the RCTs, one being a follow-up study [7]. Results of these three RCTs were published in several papers [13–15, 17, 18], but for the purpose of this review the results are summarized in three studies in Table 9.1. All studies on stroke patients were assessor blinded. The studies were typically small with <17 patients in each comparison group. Three studies included women and one included men (Table 9.1). The studies compared PFMT with standard care or general rehabilitation for stroke. In Tibaek et al.'s studies [13–15, 17, 18], the participants were exercising for 3 months, while the intervention period in Shin's study lasted 6 weeks [16]. Dropout was generally low, but adherence was not as reported in most studies. In all studies, the patients have had individual assessment of ability to contract and PFM function (manometry and/or sEMG) and close follow-up by a physical therapist in addition to a home training program. Two of the studies found statistically significant differences between groups while two did not (Table 9.1).

9.3.2 MS

Eight RCTs were found on PFMT for MS from 1997 till 2016 (Table 9.2). The studies came out from five different research groups [19–27]. One study was written in French, with only the abstract in English [25]. Five of the studies were assessor blinded, while three were not. The studies differ in sample size with a range of 10–40 in the comparison groups. All studies except one [19] included women only. One study did not report on gender (Table 9.2). Dropout was generally low, but reached 22% in two studies [22–24]. Adherence to the intervention protocol was seldom reported. In all studies, individual assessment of PFM function was assessed, mostly by vaginal palpation. Most studies compared different methods and combinations of PFMT with and without biofeedback and electrical stimulation. Two RCTs compared PFMT or combinations of PFMT and electrical stimulation with usual care/untreated control group [19, 22]. One study compared PFMT with sham training (insertion of a vaginal device, but with no contractions) [23, 24]. All the three RCTs with non-treated control groups found statistically significant improvement in outcome measures in favor of the PFMT group.

9.4 Discussion

As expected, there were fewer RCTs on the effect of PFMT in neurogenic patients compared with studies in the general population; only four and eight RCTs were found in patients with stroke and MS, respectively. No RCTs were found on patients with Parkinson's disease. Most of the studies were blinded and had low dropouts, but many had small samples sizes which could make type II error plausible when not finding statistically significant results. In addition, the studies are heterogeneous in the population studied, age of participants, methods to diagnose UI including lack of report of type of UI, use of outcome measures, and type of interventions used to treat UI. Furthermore, few research groups reported adherence, and we therefore do not know whether the participants followed the prescribed interventions. These flaws make comparison and conclusion across studies impossible. Given these limitations of the published studies, still the overall trend is that PFMT with or without combinations of other methods has a potential to improve UI in patients with stroke and MS. To date it appears to be more RCTs and stronger evidence for PFMT in patients with MS compared to patients with stroke.

The recently updated NICE guidelines [3] recommend to consider PFMT for people with lower urinary tract dysfunction due to MS or stroke or other neurological conditions where the potential to voluntarily contract the pelvic floor is preserved. They highlight that patients should be selected after specialist pelvic floor assessment and that PFMT can be considered to be combined with biofeedback and/ or electrical stimulation of the pelvic floor. Timed voiding, bladder retraining, or habit retraining can be considered for people with neurogenic lower urinary tract dysfunction to improve bladder storage, but only after assessment by a healthcare professional trained in the assessment of people with neurogenic lower urinary tract dysfunction. They also recommend that this should be done in conjunction with education about lower urinary tract function for the person and/or their family members and carers [3].

Given the few RCTs in neurologic patients there is a huge need for further high-quality research. This would imply large, possibly multicenter, RCTs with report of the effect on type of UI (SUI, UUI, and MUI) using responsive, reliable, and valid outcome measures and with a training protocol based on a theoretical framework for how this could work either for SUI [5] or OAB symptoms [7].

As to date there is no consensus on the most effective conservative treatment protocol, clinicians should follow general recommendations for PFMT and electrical stimulation shown in RCTs with statistically significant results (see references in tables of this chapter) over control and adjust this to the needs of each individual patient. If the aim is to strengthen the PFM, 3 sets of 8–12 close to maximum contractions per day for 3–6 months with weekly supervised training have shown to be effective [1, 2, 28].

For inhibition of urgency and UUI, there are less evident protocols, but most likely this also includes strengthening the PFM in order to make an inhibition of the detrusor possible. In addition, it seems important to train this inhibition during lifetime situations where urgency to void occurs [7]. All of these techniques imply a proper assessment of a healthcare provider of the patients' ability to perform a correct PFM contraction and the strength of this contraction. Assessment of ability to contract can be done with vaginal or rectal palpation, manometry, dynamometry, or ultrasonography. PFM strength is best assessed by manometry and dynamometry [29].

References

1. Dumoulin C, Cacciari LP, Hay-Smith EJC. Pelvic floor muscle training versus no treatment, or inactive control treatments, for urinary incontinence in women. Cochrane Database Syst Rev. 2018;(10):CD005654. https://doi.org/10.1002/14651858.
2. Dumoulin C, Adewuyi T, Booth J, Bradley C, Burgio B, Hagen S, Hunter K, Imamura M, Morin M, Morkved S, Thakar R, Wallace S, Williams K. Adult conservative management. In: Abrams P, Cardozo L, Wagg A, Wein A, editors. Incontinence, vol. 2. 6th ed; 2017. p. 1443–628.
3. www.NICE.guidelines. National institute for health guidelines. Urinary incontinence and urinary incontinence in neurological disease. 2019.
4. Anderson CA, Omar MI, Campbell SE, Hunter KF, Cody JD, Glazener CMA. Conservative management for postprostatectomy urinary incontinence. Cochrane Database Syst Rev. 2015;(1):CD001843. https://doi.org/10.1002/14651858.CD001843.pub5.
5. Bø K. Pelvic floor muscle training is effective in treatment of female stress urinary incontinence, but how does it work? Int Urogynecol J. 2004;15:76–84. https://doi.org/10.1007/s00192-004-1125-0.
6. Hoff Brækken IH, Majida M, Ellström Engh M, Bø K. Morphological changes after pelvic floor muscle training measured by 3-dimensional ultrasonography. A randomized controlled trial. Obstet Gynecol. 2010;115:317–24.
7. Bø K. Pelvic floor muscle training for overactive bladder. In: Bø K, Berghmans B, Mørkved S, Van Kampen M, editors. Physical therapy for the pelvic floor. Bridging science and clinical practice. 2nd ed. London: Churchill Livingstone Elsevier; 2015. p. 192–6. Chapter 7.2. Overactive bladder.
8. Shafik A, Shafik IA. Overactive bladder inhibition in response to pelvic floor muscle exercises. World J Urol. 2003;20:374–7.
9. Milsom I, Altman D, Cartwright R, Lapitan MCM, Nelson R, Sjöström S, Tikkinen KAO. Epidemiology of urinary incontinence (UI) and other lower urinary tract symptoms (LUTS), pelvic organ prolapse (POP) and anal (AI) incontinence. In: Abrams L, Wagg A, Wein A, editors. Incontinence, vol. 1. Tokyo: 6th International Consultation on Incontinence; 2017. p. 1–141.
10. Van Kampen M, Geraerts I. Evidence for pelvic floor physical therapy for neurological diseases. In: Bø K, Berghmans B, Mørkved S, Van Kampen M, editors. Chapter 12: Physical therapy for the pelvic floor. Bridging science and clinical practice. 2nd ed. London: Churchill Livingstone Elsevier; 2015. p. 387–96.
11. Hajebrahimi S, Chapple CR, Pashazadeh F, Salehi-Pourmehr H. Management of neurogenic bladder in patients with Parkinson's disease: a systematic review. Neurourol Urodyn. 2019;38(1):31–62. https://doi.org/10.1002/nau.23991.
12. Thomas H, Cross S, Barrett J, French B, Leathley M, Sutton CJ, Watkins C. Treatment of urinary incontinence after stroke in adults. Cochrane Database Syst Rev. 2008;(1):CD004462.
13. Tibaek S, Jensen R, Lindskov G, Jensen M. Can quality of life be improved by pelvic floor muscle training in women with urinary incontinence after ischemic stroke? A randomised controlled and blinded study. Int Urogynecol J. 2004;15:117–23.
14. Tibaek S, Gard G, Jensen R. Pelvic floor muscle training is effective in women with urinary incontinence after stroke. A randomised controlled and blinded study. Neurourol Urodyn. 2005;24:348–57.
15. Tibaek S, Gard G, Jensen R. Is there a long-lasting effect of pelvic floor muscle training in women with urinary incontinence after ischemic stroke? Int Urogynecol J. 2007;18:281–7.
16. Shin DC, Shin SH, Lee MM, Lee KJ, Song CH. Pelvic floor muscle training for urinary incontinence in female stroke patients: a randomized controlled and blinded trial. Clin Rehabil. 2016;30:259–67.
17. Tibaek S, Gard G, Dehlendorff C, Iversen HK, Biering-Soerensen F, Jensen R. Is pelvic floor muscle training effective for men with poststroke lower urinary tract symptoms? A single – blinded randomized controlled trial. Am J Mens Health. 2007;11:1460–71.

18. Tibaek S, Gard G, Dehlendorff C, Iversen HK, Bjering-Soerensen F, Jensen R. Can pelvic floor muscle training improve quality of life in men with mild to moderate post-stroke and lower urinary tract symptoms? Eur J Phys Rehabil Med. 2016;53:416–25.
19. Vahtera T, Haaranen M, Viramo-Koskela AL, et al. Pelvic floor rehabilitation is effective in patients with multiple sclerosis. Clin Rehabil. 1997;11:211–9.
20. McClurg D, Ashe RG, Marshall K, Lowe-Strong AS. Comparison of pelvic floor muscle training, electromyography biofeedback, and neuromuscular electrical stimulation for bladder dysfunction in people with multiple sclerosis: a randomized pilot study. Neurourol Urodyn. 2006;25:337–48.
21. McClurg D, Ashe RG, Lowe-Strong AS. Neuromuscular electrical stimulation and the treatment of lower urinary tract dysfunction in multiple sclerosis. A double blind, placebo controlled, randomized clinical trial. Neurourol Urodyn. 2008;27:231–7.
22. Khan F, Pallant JF, Pallant JI, Brand C, Kilpatrick TJ. A randomised controlled trial: outcomes of bladder rehabilitation in persons with multiple sclerosis. J Neurol Neurosurg Psychiatry. 2010;81:1033–8.
23. Lucio AC, Campos RM, Perissinoto MC, Miyaoka R, Damasceno BP, D'ancona CA. Pelvic floor muscle training in the treatment of urinary tract symptoms in women with multiple sclerosis. Neurourol Urodyn. 2010;29:1410–3.
24. Lucio AC, Perissinoto MC, Natalin RA, Prudente A, Damasceno BP, D'ancona CA. A comparative study of pelvic floor muscle training in women with multiple sclerosis: its impact on lower urinary tract symptoms and quality of life. Clinics. 2011;66:1563–8.
25. Gaspard L, Tombai B, Opsomer RJ, Castille Y, Van Pesch V, Detrembleur C. Physiotherapy and neurogenic lower urinary tract dysfunction in multiple sclerosis patients: a randomized controlled trial. Prog Urol. 2014;24:697–707.
26. Ferreira APS, Pegorare AMGS, Salgodo PR, Casafus FS, Christifoletti G. Impact of a pelvic floor muscle training program among women with multiple sclerosis. A controlled clinical trial. Am J Phys Med Rehabil. 2016;95:1–8.
27. Lucio A, D'ancona CA, Perissinptto MC, McLean L, Damasceno BP, de Moraes Lopes MH. Pelvic floor muscle training with and without electrical stimulation in the treatment of lower urinary tract symptoms in women with multiple sclerosis. J Wound Ostomy Continence Nurs. 2016;43:414–9.
28. Bø K, Aschehoug A. Strength training. In: Bø K, Berghmans B, Mørkved S, Van Kampen M, editors. Physical therapy for the pelvic floor. Bridging science and clinical practice. 2nd ed. London: Churchill Livingstone Elsevier; 2015. p. 111–30. Chapter 6. Pelvic floor and exercise science.
29. Bø K, Sherburn M. Evaluation of female pelvic-floor muscle function and strength. Phys Ther. 2005;85:269–82.

Sexual Dysfunction in Suprapontine Lesions

David B. Vodušek

Sexuality is a component of a fulfilled life. Neurologic disease may affect the sexual function by the neural lesion itself, or by its treatment, but also because of other disease-related deficits and issues including psychosocial and cultural changes resulting from the chronic disease.

Loss of sexual desire (or hypersexuality), erectile and ejaculatory dysfunction in men, decreased lubrication in women, and disturbances of orgasm are more common in neurological patients than in the general population, but are often not communicated by them to their doctor. Sexual symptoms may be relevant for the diagnosis, significantly affect the quality of life, and may be responsive to treatment.

10.1 Sexual Function and the Nervous System

The sexual response is traditionally conceptualized as a sequence of phases, desire, arousal, and orgasm, but it can also be seen as a cycle of overlapping phases, more appropriate for the description of the female sexual response [1]. In any case, sexual behavior involves a series of neurally controlled phenomena including normal vasculature, occurring in a hormonally defined milieu.

The primary sensory areas in the brain and the parietal and inferior temporal lobes process sexual stimuli; the forebrain regulates the initiation and the execution of sexual behavior; the medial preoptic area integrates sensory and hormonal signals; and the amygdala plays a role in the reward aspects of sexual function. Neurons from the paraventricular nucleus project to the thoracic and lumbosacral spinal cord

D. B. Vodušek (✉)
Division of Neurology, Institute for Clinical Neurophysiology, University Medical Centre Ljubljana, Ljubljana, Slovenia
e-mail: david.vodusek@kclj.si

© Springer Nature Switzerland AG 2020
G. Lamberti et al. (eds.), *Suprapontine Lesions and Neurogenic Pelvic Dysfunctions*, Urodynamics, Neurourology and Pelvic Floor Dysfunctions,
https://doi.org/10.1007/978-3-030-29775-6_10

nuclei, which, by way of the sympathetic, parasympathetic, and somatic nerves, affect the genital response [2]. Fertility and procreation are importantly linked to sexuality, but will not be discussed here.

10.2   Change in Sexual Function with Aging

When examining the sexuality of neurological patients, their premorbid status has to be ascertained.

In the elderly the frequency of intercourse as a rule decreases and sexual dysfunction is more prevalent than in younger patients; nevertheless, about a quarter of those aged 75–85 years report sexual activity. Males need more time and stimuli to achieve erection and orgasm, and their refractory period after detumescence is prolonged. In the female, there is decreased libido and thinning of the vaginal wall with decreased elasticity and lubrication [3].

10.3   Evaluation of Patients with Sexual Dysfunction and Neurologic Disorders

The history reveals the relevant sexual symptoms, and other factors influencing sexual functioning, including drugs. Formal questionnaires can be used to obtain standardized information on male and female sexual function.

On clinical examination changes in pigmentation and body hair, and presence of galactorrhea, should be noted. Functional investigations of genital arousal are not performed, unless vasogenic erectile dysfunction is suspected (in men). Neurophysiological testing may clarify the topical diagnosis only in infrapontine lesions. Patients with suspected endocrine dysfunction should be referred to the endocrinologist.

10.4   Sexual Dysfunction in Patients with Suprapontine Lesions

In patients with suprapontine lesions the prevalence of sexual dysfunction is reportedly higher than in the general population, but few epidemiological studies have been done.

10.4.1 Head and Brain Injuries

Some cognitive impairment, personality change, and sensorimotor disability often remain after traumatic brain injury and may be accompanied by sexual dysfunction. Among patients with closed-head injury admitted for 24 h or more, significant sexual dysfunction was found in 50% over a 15-year time span.

Frontal and temporal lesions seem to result more often in sexual disturbances than parieto-occipital lesions. Symptoms may occur, at least in part, as a consequence of posttraumatic pituitary dysfunction [4].

Hypersexuality, disinhibited and inappropriate sexual behavior, sexually aggressive behavior, and changes in sexual preference sometimes follow basal frontal and limbic brain injury and may lead to sex offences. Bilateral anterior temporal lesions result in the Klüver–Bucy syndrome with hypersexuality and pansexuality [5].

10.4.2 Hypothalamopituitary Disorders

Hypothalamopituitary dysfunction is usually caused by a pituitary adenoma. Three-fourths of patients have decreased or absent libido at the time of diagnosis. Erectile dysfunction is common, but because of reduced sexual interest is less distressing.

Most female patients have amenorrhea. Women with hypoprolactinemia complain of loss of sexual desire [6].

10.4.3 Cerebrovascular Disease

About 75% of patients who were sexually active before the stroke report a subsequent decrease in coital frequency. Late outcome studies are scant; poor sexual functioning may persist even with otherwise good improvement. Many men (up to 65%) have erectile dysfunction after a stroke; orgasmic and ejaculatory dysfunction are common. Decreased vaginal lubrication and inability to achieve orgasm occur in female patients. Function may, however, return within a year.

Patients and their partners may avoid sexual intercourse out of concern of recurrence. The workload during sexual activity is similar to that of climbing stairs or walking briskly. Although the exact risk of stroke during sexual activity is not known, it seems to be low. Patients and their partners may thus be reassured that, in resuming sexual activity, the gains in most instances outweigh any slight risks.

Hypersexuality after stroke has been described, but seems to be rare [7].

10.4.4 Parkinsonism and Basal Ganglia Disorders

The dopaminergic system is intimately involved in neural circuits controlling desire and arousal. Patients with Parkinson's disease of both genders show a decrease in libido, in frequency of intercourse, and in the ability to reach orgasm. In men, erection and ejaculation may be affected. In women, vaginal tightness and involuntary urination during intercourse are reported.

Muscle rigidity and bradykinesia may impair sexual activity; tremor may be enhanced during sexual arousal. All these may be worse in the late evenings if dose scheduling is aimed at favoring daytime activities.

Dopaminergic treatment may result in an apparent increase, or normalization, of libido even without corresponding improvement in motor symptoms. Spontaneous erections have been reported in patients receiving levodopa and dopaminergic agonists. About 3% of treated patients demonstrate true hypersexuality.

Deep brain stimulation of the subthalamic nucleus may have a positive influence on sexual well-being of men, but hypersexuality has also been reported [8].

In multiple system atrophy, erectile dysfunction usually begins several years before the onset of other neurologic symptoms. By the time of diagnosis, 30% of patients were also unable to ejaculate. Patients of both genders have a decrease in desire and the ability to reach orgasm, and the frequency of intercourse falls. Hypersexuality may occur with dopaminergic treatment.

Approximately 10% of patients with Huntington disease have increased sexual activity, sometimes associated with mania or hypomania. Promiscuity may be an early or initial symptom of the disease. But patients also report difficulties in becoming sexually aroused. Paraphilias such as sexual aggression, exhibitionism, and pedophilia occur.

Disinhibited sexual behavior is common in patients with Gilles de la Tourette syndrome [9].

10.4.5 Multiple Sclerosis

Sexual dysfunction affects eventually the majority of patients and decreases their quality of life.

Erectile dysfunction is rare initially, but becomes more common with the evolution of multiple sclerosis. Spontaneous improvement sometimes occurs. Problems with ejaculation are frequent and are often coupled to the erectile dysfunction.

Decreased vaginal lubrication and sensory disturbances involving the genital region (hypoesthesia, hyperesthesia, and different types of pain) are common and may be apparent already in the early stages of multiple sclerosis. Sacral-segment dysesthesias may be so severe that patients are unable to bear direct genital contact.

Decreased libido but also hypersexuality may occur.

Other symptoms related to multiple sclerosis, such as fatigue, depression, cognitive dysfunction, spasticity in the lower limbs, urinary and bowel disturbances, and use of aids to manage incontinence, can inhibit sexuality, as can paroxysmal motor and sensory disturbances, triggered by sexual intercourse [10].

10.4.6 Epilepsy

Epilepsy is associated with sexual problems, more often in men than women. It is helpful to determine whether disturbances relate to seizures or occur during the interictal period.

Hyperventilation accompanying sexual activity can provoke generalized epileptic seizures. Sexual fantasies as well as genital stimuli (masturbation) or orgasm may trigger reflex epilepsy.

Sensations in the genital organs may be manifestations of a partial epileptic seizure arising from a genital sensory cortical area. Motor symptoms such as erection and ejaculation or the sensory experience of an orgasm may also occur, the latter particularly from right mesio-temporal foci. Pelvic sexual movements, as a part of epileptic automatisms, or compulsive masturbation in front of others may occur during or after a seizure. Such events may be experienced by patients as sexual or nonsexual.

Complex sexual experiences occur most often in patients with temporal lobe lesions. Sexual automatisms may also occur with frontal lobe lesions.

Interictally, loss of sexual desire, reduced sexual activity, or inhibited sexual arousal are reported. Sexual interest is more reduced in patients with left temporal lobe lesions. Paranoid delusions of a sexual nature occur in some.

Antiepileptic drugs, especially older agents (phenytoin, phenobarbital, primidone, carbamazepine, and valproate), lead to hormonal changes (particularly increased estradiol and decreased free testosterone levels in men), and decreased sexual desire and performance in both sexes. The effect of the newer anticonvulsant drugs on sexual function is claimed to be less. Restoration of sexual function has been reported after successful surgery for epilepsy [11].

10.5 Treatment of Sexual Dysfunction

Sexual dysfunction associated with neurologic disease often increases patients' distress. Discussion with patients and partners about their sexual life should be part of any rehabilitation strategy. In all instances, drug regimens should be reviewed for possible effects on sexual function. Sexual education, counseling, and specific suggestions about therapeutic methods are important, and should be provided by the treating physician. In a limited number of patients, referral to a sexual therapist may be indicated. Methods for sexual rehabilitation in the context of neurologic disorders have been described [12].

10.5.1 Treatment of Neurogenic Erectile Dysfunction

The development of drug treatments by the oral and intracavernous routes has revolutionized the outlook for men with erectile failure. The selective inhibitors of type 5 cyclic guanosine monophosphate phosphodiesterase augment the nitric oxide-mediated relaxation pathway in penile tissues by increasing available cyclic guanosine monophosphate in the corpus cavernosum. These medications therefore do not cause erection but enhance the response to sexual arousal. Sildenafil taken at bedtime also significantly increases nocturnal erections.

Sildenafil is an effective treatment for erectile dysfunction in neurological patients; good studies have been done in patients with multiple sclerosis [13] and with Parkinson's disease (cf 8), but experience supports the use of this (and similar) medicine in all neurological patients.

Sildenafil (25, 50, or 100 mg) can be taken orally 1 h before intended sexual activity. (Significant effects have been reported between 30 min and 4–6 h after taking the medication.) It should be noted that a meal delays absorption of the drug, and so does slowed gastric emptying such as seen in Parkinson's disease and autonomic neuropathy. Treatment should be begun with 25–50 mg, and the same dose taken several times before it is increased. Dose-finding studies have demonstrated a dose-response curve. Sildenafil can be used repeatedly, and if used once or twice per week there should be no fear of tachyphylaxis.

Phosphodiesterase-5 inhibitors are contraindicated in combination with vasodilator drugs of the nitro type and nitric oxide donors, but a cardiologist can change such drug regimens in suitable patients with erectile difficulties requiring treatment. Phosphodiesterase-5 inhibitors should not be used in patients with retinitis pigmentosa. They are contraindicated in men with hypotension (blood pressure below 90/50 mmHg). Care should be taken to identify men with multiple system atrophy who may have erectile dysfunction, atypical parkinsonism, and asymptomatic postural hypotension. In our experience, an intelligent patient can use sildenafil after clear explanation, with careful planning of activity during the several hours after drug intake and performing sexual activity in the recumbent position.

No evidence was found of sildenafil effects on the myocardium or the conduction system. However, evaluation of functional capacity is necessary in patients with coronary artery disease, who need to know the risks of physical (and sexual) activity. Patients who can exercise up to 4.5 metabolic equivalents without angina or hypotension can probably use sildenafil safely. Recommendations for the use of sildenafil in patients with cardiovascular disease have been published. In controlled and open-label studies, no increased risk of cerebrovascular events has been reported.

The most common adverse events of sildenafil are headache, flushing, and dyspepsia. Temporary visual symptoms (mainly color-vision disturbances) may occur with higher doses (100 mg), and nonvasculitic anterior optic neuropathy has been described in rare instances. Adverse effects are mostly transitory and of minor intensity [14].

Treatment with apomorphine sublingually is an effective option for men with erectile dysfunction, but due to its weaker effect and obnoxious side effect (nausea) it is not available commercially in most countries.

Yohimbine is an ancient aphrodisiac which has little to offer in the presence of modern drugs [11].

10.5.2 Intracavernous Injection Therapy with Vasoactive Drugs

Prostaglandin E_1 (alprostadil) is the preferred drug for self-injection therapy in erectile dysfunction, and low doses are effective in neurogenic impotence. The effect is rapid and independent of sexual excitement and may last for 2–4 h. Local bleeding, pain, and fibrosis may develop in the corpora cavernosa, leading to loss of effectiveness. This treatment is contraindicated in patients taking anticoagulants or with hematologic malignancies.

Long-lasting erections—priapism—as an adverse drug reaction usually have a good prognosis with conservative treatment [15].

10.5.3 Other Treatment Options

With a dedicated vacuum device, rigidity adequate for penetration occurs in most patients with neurogenic erectile dysfunction. The most common complications are bruises, petechiae, and skin edema. The constriction band should not stay in place for longer than 30 min.

The use of a constriction band on its own may help patients who can obtain an erection, albeit not a durable one; the same restrictions concerning the duration of application should be observed.

In neurogenic erectile dysfunction, part of the problem may be penile sensory loss. Additional vibratory stimulation may help in producing a rigid erection sufficient for vaginal penetration.

As a last resort, surgical treatment is also possible (penile prostheses) [12].

10.5.4 Premature Ejaculation

Counseling on the use of particular techniques during coitus may lead to improvement. Pharmacotherapeutic options include antidepressants (selective serotonin reuptake inhibitors such as paroxetine), and phosphodiesterase-5 inhibitors, used off label [16].

10.5.5 Treatment in Women with Sexual Dysfunction

Vibratory stimulation and dildos may be helpful and are routinely advised in patients with genital sensory disturbances and in those with weakness or motor disorders.

In women with dysesthetic or painful sensations in the genitalia that are not alleviated by improving lubrication, antiepileptic drugs such as gabapentin, pregabalin, and carbamazepine may help. Efficacy and safety of flibanserin (with minor effects in treatment of hypoactive sexual desire syndrome) in neurogenic dysfunction are not reported.

10.5.6 Treatment of Hypersexuality

For abnormally increased libido, pharmacologic treatment should be checked. Androgen antagonists (cyproterone acetate, medroxyprogesterone acetate) may be effective. In resistant cases, neuroleptics are usually helpful [12].

10.6 Concluding Comments

Tools to define the individual role of different biologic factors (such as endocrine, neurologic, vascular, endothelial, and other factors) and of psychosocial influences in the individual with sexual dysfunction are still crude. The options to help patients have nevertheless improved significantly and help can be offered to the patient and the partner.

References

1. Basson R. Human sexual response. In: Vodušek DB, Boller F, editors. Neurology of sexual and bladder disorders. Amsterdam: Elsevier; 2015. p. 11–8.
2. Komisaruk BR, Rodriguez del Cerro MC. Human sexual behavior related to pathology and activity of the brain. In: Vodušek DB, Boller F, editors. Neurology of sexual and bladder disorders. Amsterdam: Elsevier; 2015. p. 109–20.
3. Lindau ST, Schumm LP, Laumann EO. A study of sexuality and health among older adults in the United States. N Engl J Med. 2007;357:762–74.
4. O'Carroll R, Woodrow J, Maroun F. Psychosexual and psychosocial sequelae of closed head injury. Brain Inj. 1991;5:303–13.
5. Hayman LA, Rexer JL, Pavol MA. Klüver-Bucy syndrome after bilateral selective damage of amygdala and its cortical connections. J Neuropsychiatry Clin Neurosci. 1998;10:354–8.
6. Lundberg P, Hulter B. Sexual dysfunction in patients with hypothalamo-pituitary disorders. Exp Clin Endocrinol. 1991;98:81–8.
7. Boller F, Agrawal K, Romano A. Sexual function after strokes. In: Vodušek DB, Boller F, editors. Neurology of sexual and bladder disorders. Amsterdam: Elsevier; 2015. p. 289–96.
8. Bronner G, Vodušek DB. Management of sexual dysfunction in Parkinson's disease. Ther Adv Neurol Disord. 2011;4:375–83.
9. Lombroso PJ, Scahill LD, Chappell PB. Tourette's syndrome: a multigenerational, neuropsychiatric disorder. Adv Neurol. 1995;65:305–18.
10. Lew-Starowicz M, Gianotten WL. Sexual dysfunction in patients with multiple sclerosis. In: Vodušek DB, Boller F, editors. Neurology of sexual and bladder disorders. Amsterdam: Elsevier; 2015. p. 357–70.
11. Luef G, Madersbacher H. Sexual dysfunction in patients with epilepsy. In: Vodušek DB, Boller F, editors. Neurology of sexual and bladder disorders. Amsterdam: Elsevier; 2015. p. 383–94.
12. Basson R, Bronner G. Management and rehabilitation of neurologic patients with sexual dysfunction. In: Vodušek DB, Boller F, editors. Neurology of sexual and bladder disorders. Amsterdam: Elsevier; 2015. p. 415–35.
13. Fowler CJ, Miller JR, Sharief MK, Hussain IF, Stecher VJ, Sweeney M. A double blind, randomised study of sildenafil citrate for erectile dysfunction in men with multiple sclerosis. J Neurol Neurosurg Psychiatry. 2005;76:700–5.
14. Salonia A, Rigatti P, Montorsi F. Sildenafil in erectile dysfunction: a critical review. Curr Med Res Opin. 2003;19:241–62.
15. Porst H. The rationale for prostaglandin E_1 in erectile failure: a survey of worldwide experience. J Urol. 1996;155:802–15.
16. Perelman MA. A new combination treatment for premature ejaculation: a sex therapist's perspective. J Sex Med. 2006;3:1004–12.